DATE DUE

7/11/12			

Demco

Low Income, Social Growth, and Good Health

CALIFORNIA/MILBANK BOOKS ON HEALTH AND THE PUBLIC

Low Income, Social Growth, and Good Health

A History of Twelve Countries

James C. Riley

UNIVERSITY OF CALIFORNIA PRESS
Berkeley / Los Angeles / London
MILBANK MEMORIAL FUND
New York

University of California Press, one of the most distinguished university presses in the United States, enriches lives around the world by advancing scholarship in the humanities, social sciences, and natural sciences. Its activities are supported by the UC Press Foundation and by philanthropic contributions from individuals and institutions. For more information, visit www.ucpress.edu.

University of California Press
Berkeley and Los Angeles, California

University of California Press, Ltd.
London, England

© 2008 by The Regents of the University of California

Library of Congress Cataloging-in-Publication Data

Riley, James C.
    Low income, social growth, and good health : a history of twelve countries / James C. Riley.
        p.   cm. — (California/Milbank books on health and the public ; 17)
    Includes bibliographical references and index.
    ISBN 978-0-520-25286-8 (cloth : alk. paper)
        1. Life expectancy—Economic aspects—Case studies.   I. Milbank Memorial Fund.   II. Title.   III. Series.

HB1322.3.R54   2007
304.6'45—dc22   2007004611

Manufactured in the United States of America

16   15   14   13   12   11   10   09   08
10   9   8   7   6   5   4   3   2   1

This book is printed on New Leaf EcoBook 50, a 100% recycled fiber of which 50% is de-inked post-consumer waste, processed chlorine-free. EcoBook 50 is acid-free and meets the minimum requirements of ANSI/ASTM D5634–01 (*Permanence of Paper*).

For Valin

Contents

Illustrations

Tables

Figures

Foreword

The Milbank Memorial Fund is an endowed operating foundation that works to improve health by helping decision makers in the public and private sectors acquire and use the best available evidence to inform policy for health care and population health. The Fund has engaged in nonpartisan analysis, study, research, and communication on significant issues in health policy since its inception in 1905.

Low Income, Social Growth, and Good Health: A History of Twelve Countries is the seventeenth of the California / Milbank Books on Health and the Public. The publishing partnership between the Fund and the University of California Press seeks to encourage the synthesis and communication of findings from research that could contribute to more effective health policy.

James C. Riley's research makes him a critic of the high priority accorded to economic growth by most national and multilateral development agencies. In the twelve countries he studied for this book, increased life expectancy and healthier populations were the basis for rather than the result of economic growth. People had longer and healthier lives in these countries because of "social growth" that enabled even poor communities to organize programs of schooling, public health, and health care.

Unlike most analysts and critics of policy for aid to low-income countries, Riley uses the methods of social history and historical epidemiology. He draws his generalizations from case studies of the attainment of increased life expectancy during the twentieth century in twelve countries in very different regions of the world.

Unlike wealthy countries, whose history in the nineteenth century has been the model for most development policy, each of the countries Riley studied "managed to initiate and sustain social growth from a position of near poverty." Wealthy countries, he writes, "used rising levels of income in the hands of consumers and government to pay for social growth." By contrast, the countries Riley presents and assesses "found ways to build their own forms of social capital," especially primary schools, health care, and public health services, including educating their citizens about the "health risks they faced and how to temper them."

Riley's research also suggests that there is no template for policy that can be applied in every low-income country. In an earlier book, *Rising Life Expectancy: A Global History*, he assessed the influence of six variables on reduced mortality: public health; medicine; wealth, income and economic development; famine, malnutrition and diet; household and individual behavior; and literacy and education. The evidence in this book strengthens the finding of his earlier research that "different countries and different populations have used different combinations" of programs to achieve lower mortality.

Riley's central message is that, rather than seek a "leading or dominant explanation of social or economic growth" as the "marker for countries that lag," scholars and policymakers should be more attentive to programs that are "most easily adopted in the circumstances that prevail" in each low-income country. He urges leaders of donor organizations to shift their emphasis from development policy that encourages substantial innovation in public policy and individual behavior to "finding the adaptations that can most readily be made [in a country] given existing patterns of behavior, habits of mind, institutions, [and] resources."

Daniel M. Fox
President

Samuel L. Milbank
Chairman

Preface and Acknowledgments

By the early years of the twenty-first century all the high-income countries of the world had attained life expectancies at birth within the range 76.1 (Portugal) to 81.5 years (Japan).[1] More surprisingly, a significant number of middle- and low-income countries had also attained life expectancies within this range or close to it. Economic development indeed has led to better survival: the high-income countries all share high life expectancies, although most of those countries attained their position gradually, across decades of effort. There have, however, been other paths to high survival as well. This book explores how twelve countries improved survival prospects either without becoming rich lands or before becoming rich lands.

Students trying to understand how populations arrive at good survival and high life expectancy have often tried to explain the present from the present, rather than from past experience merging into the present. To understand how a country attained its current position, it is essential to consider circumstances before and during the period when sustained gains in survival began, and then onward through those gains. In following that approach, this book demonstrates that income becomes just one candidate factor to explain gains in survival.

Most of the help I received in doing research for this book came from two sources, the first being fellow scholars who suggested material to read on the history of mortality in individual countries and the second being librarians who helped me obtain that and other relevant material. For the first type of assistance I want to thank Jonathan Brown, Ben Eklof,

Zadia M. Feliciano, Randy Hanson, Hiroaki Kuromiya, Chris Langford, John Lombardi, Ethan Michelson, Cormac Ó Gráda, Steven Palmer, Sam Preston, and K. A. P. Siddhisena. For the second kind of assistance I thank the many people who played a part in building the magnificent research collections of modern times, among them especially the librarians at Indiana University.

Indiana University provided a research stipend. Allan G. Hill, José M. Avilán Rovira, and Tai-Hun Kim helped me obtain material I would not otherwise have been able to consult. Walter Nugent deserves special thanks for suggesting that I work on this topic. For critical comments on earlier drafts I thank José M. Avilán Rovira, Stan Engerman, Dan Fox, Steve Kunitz, Massimo Livi Bacci, and Walter Nugent. For help on later drafts I want to thank the following referees selected by the Milbank Memorial Fund and the University of California Press: Jack Caldwell, Bruce Fetter, Godfrey Gunatilleke, Stephen Leeder, and Kenneth Prewitt. At the Press Lynne Withey, Hannah Love, and their colleagues made the publication process comfortable as well as professional. My copyeditor, Ellen F. Smith, did a wonderful job. I am grateful to all these people.

Bloomington, June 2007

Introduction

Living into old age is the prize, much more so than being rich or surrounded by material possessions, although some people would add a qualifier: living into old age in acceptable health. Yet even though people treasure health and survival, they direct their life efforts—they scheme and plan—more often toward material prosperity than toward preserving health and attaining old age. The same thing has been true of nations.

Nations have sought explicitly to make themselves rich much more aggressively than they have sought to make their populations long-lived. The first instances of sustained economic growth appeared in Britain and Belgium in the last decades of the eighteenth century and early decades of the nineteenth century. By 1960 fifteen or twenty countries had found their own paths to sustained growth and become rich lands. And by that date nearly every other country around the globe had set this target as its chief objective. Individuals believed that they could become as rich as their counterparts in the most favored countries, such as the United States. National leaders believed they could identify and implement policies that would make their countries rich. And international agencies, chief among them the World Bank, believed they could provide the advice and the credit essential to transform the globe from poverty to riches.

The confidence felt by all these groups in the 1950s and 1960s turned out to be unwarranted. A few countries have since become rich, and a larger number have broken out of the ranks of poor lands into a new territory of middle-income counties. Yet much more was hoped in the way of economic growth than now, early in the twenty-first century, has been achieved. In some countries people gained higher incomes but did not manage to initiate sustained economic growth; in many other countries people sank into deeper poverty, or at best found themselves still relatively impoverished while a few fellow citizens joined a rich elite. Nevertheless, nearly everyone has sustained the hope that people everywhere can become rich, or at least enough better off to escape day-to-day anxieties about providing themselves with basic necessities of life and giving their children the means to live to another day.

As the record to be examined here will suggest, there was another possibility among the choices that might have been made in the 1950s and 1960s about where to invest our hopes, our planning, and our scheming. Individuals, leaders, and internationalist givers of credit and advice might have elected instead to focus on health and survival, and on the things that build health and survival in nations. If they had done that, they would have looked not so closely at the experience of Britain as the first industrial nation or at how other countries managed in the nineteenth century to initiate sustained economic growth. They would have looked instead at the countries where people lived into old age. By 1960 that group included all the countries that had become rich. Those rich lands and the householders in them used some of the benefits of material prosperity to protect themselves from hazards to their health. They built hospitals; they trained doctors and nurses; they purified water and delivered it in pipes to people's homes while removing human waste in a parallel system of pipes and sewers; and they accumulated a vast body of learning about disease and its prevention and treatment. Because they were rich countries, they could spend generously on health, even though that was an afterthought to becoming rich.

But another group of countries might also have drawn attention. For among those countries where people lived to old age were poor lands that had nevertheless managed to initiate health transitions, that is, gains in life expectancy that were sustained and that carried the population from circumstances in which the most common age at death was infancy to those in which most people lived into old age. Being poor, these countries and most of the people in them could not afford to follow the path the rich lands had taken to high life expectancy: it was too costly. They had to discover a path of their own, one their inhabitants could afford.

How this group of low-income countries managed to make such rapid and sustained gains in survival, mostly between 1920 and 1960, that they matched the rich countries in life expectancy is the subject of this book.

What distinguishes these countries is that they managed to initiate and sustain social growth from a position of near poverty. The high-income countries used rising levels of income in the hands of consumers and governments to pay for social growth, building schools and training teachers, expanding public health facilities, training health care providers, introducing pensions, disability payments, maternal and child health care, and, in most cases, establishing health care systems paid for out of public revenues. Those things constituted *social capital* in the form of physical assets plus human knowledge and skills.

The countries investigated in this book built social capital in a different way, one that represents a form of development peculiar to low-income countries. Through the pursuit of what is called *social growth* or *social development,* rather than economic development, low-income countries found ways to build their own forms of social capital even though their people had little capacity for spending on things other than the basic necessities of life and their governments lacked the revenues to fund costly programs. For the most part these countries did not try, in their key period of social growth from 1920 to 1960, to establish programs of publicly funded welfare, unemployment compensation, pensions, or housing subsidies. They concentrated instead on primary schools, public health, and health care. Because they could not afford simply to buy these things, their task was to engage the community in a collaborative effort to build and use them. These countries displayed a preference for social growth and the accumulation of social capital in five particular areas: public health; education; basic health care; the people's understanding of the health risks they faced and how to temper them; and the people's participation in the effort to improve their own lives and their own survival.

In this sense, therefore, social capital refers to some physical improvements, including primary schools and clinics; to community learning about how to combat leading health risks; and to a household-level effort to improve health. The key elements were primary schooling, the dissemination of information about disease hazards and how to avoid them, and engagement of ordinary people in controlling disease risks.

The idea that individuals need to be attuned to the health risks associated with diet and some behaviors, such as cigarette smoking, is a commonplace in Western countries in the face of today's profile of causes of death, which is led by chronic organ diseases. This investigation will show that individual and household-level understanding of health risks also mattered in the era of communicable diseases. Education in the characteristics of important communicable diseases, how to recognize them, and how to reduce chances of becoming sick played a prominent part in early reductions in mortality in low-income countries.

Many countries tried in the 1950s and have tried since then, often with advice, aid, and loans from the West, to initiate economic growth without building social capital in the ways identified here. They have, in effect, tried to skip a step in the process of development, and they have assumed, along with their advisers, that a better quality of life for their people, including better survival for infants, children, and adults, would follow once economic development had been successfully launched. They have believed also that the wonder drugs, the antibiotics introduced in the 1940s and 1950s, the new vaccines of the 1950s and 1960s, and later medical innovations might make the accumulation of social capital unnecessary, and that drugs, vaccines, and medical innovations could be sufficient to defeat the three great scourges of humankind: fecal disease, malaria, and tuberculosis.

Like today's high-income countries, however, the countries studied here brought these diseases under control before the introduction of DDT, antibiotics, and the new vaccines. In other words, they initiated health transitions and made rapid gains in life expectancy without relying on modern medical technology.

The history of health and survival in high-income lands shows that economic growth can provide the resources for a health transition. The history of health and survival in the low-income countries under study here shows that social growth can achieve the same thing. The case studies assembled in this book suggest that trying to initiate economic growth as a foundation for a higher standard of living and for longer lives has proved, because of the difficulty of moving all the world onto the path of becoming rich, to be a mistake. What is essential, at least for longer lives, is to build social capital.

Earlier Studies of Low-Income Countries with Good Health

Students of health and survival began in the 1970s to notice that some low-income countries had attained life expectancy at or close to the level in the rich lands, and to wonder how that had been done. The first case that came to wide attention was the state of Kerala in India.[1] Even though Kerala was one of the poorer states in a poor land, the life expectancy of its residents far surpassed that of other states in India.

This issue gained wider notice in the 1980s as more cases were noticed, and an explanatory theory began to emerge. Not just Kerala state but also Sri Lanka and Costa Rica drew attention as poor lands with good health. The first argument made was that these countries had achieved good health by emphasizing social justice rather than economic growth.[2] Under policies inspired by the premise of social justice, these lands elected to distribute access to health care, education, and food equitably while also providing greater autonomy for women. In primary schooling these lands provided spaces for girls as well as boys; in households women joined in decision-making about family matters, especially regarding the children; and in the wider community women took a serious part in decision-making.

In the same decade a team of experts assembled by the Rockefeller Foundation examined China, Kerala state, Sri Lanka, and Costa Rica under the theme "good health at low cost," which was the title given the collection of essays that these experts produced.[3] Working at a moment of high hopes for primary health care, the team noticed in all four cases that people had ready access to health care, to barefoot doctors in China and to numerous and accessible clinics in Sri Lanka, Costa Rica, and Kerala state. The experts considered other explanations, too. One expert emphasized the importance of adequate nutrition, education, and a group of interventions: vaccines, oral rehydration therapy for diarrhea, family planning, and primary health care. To create and implement those things, this expert suggested that a population needed both a marked degree of self-reliance and a commitment to social reciprocity, in which people treated one another with dignity. Members of the team pointed up the different paths followed by the four countries. Another researcher found the basis of success in political and social will. The team as a whole settled on three leading factors: broad access to public health and primary health care, backed up by more specialized health facilities; education; and adequate nutrition.

About a decade later the United Nations Research Institute for Social Development decided to underwrite a research project that aimed to improve "understanding of the reasons behind the superior social performance of some developing countries, and to reveal conditions under which social progress can occur independently of economic advance" by examining seven successful cases. Like earlier researchers, the participants in this project considered Costa Rica, Kerala, and Sri Lanka. They added China, Cuba, Vietnam, and Chile, and mentioned Jamaica, Argentina, and Uruguay as cases that might also have been considered. Although a plurality of the countries examined might have been singled out for the opportunities they offered girls and women and for their attachment to social justice policies, the participants found quite another set of explanations. "Three common factors have been crucial to . . . success," they stated: "political leadership committed to extending vital social services to the entire population"; political systems, whether democratic or authoritarian, that invested in social development; and "strong action by the public sector in the provision of certain health and education services," which itself was allied to development of "the administrative capacity of the state and the infrastructure to reach all parts of the country."[4] What mattered, they argued, was less the proportion of expenditures devoted to health and education and more the administrative capacity to execute a design once articulated.

UNICEF, too, joined this effort by supporting a research project that broadened the issue to ask why some countries have social indicators in general, not just in mortality, that far surpass what would be expected from their level of income. The UNICEF team likewise considered Costa Rica, Kerala, and Sri Lanka, but added Cuba, Barbados, Botswana, Zimbabwe, Mauritius, the Republic of Korea, and Malaysia—a mixed group of which about half combined rapid and sustained economic growth with social development. This team found many routes to social development, low mortality, and educational attainment but some important commonalities in social and economic policies. In this study too, the state played a preeminent role in ensuring that most people had access to basic social services. Their answer focuses on the importance of "public action for social development."[5]

Like the other early participants in this discussion, contributors to the UN Research Institute for Social Development and UNICEF projects tried to explain the achievements of good health at low cost by examining the period from the 1960s to the 1990s. The UNICEF team insisted on the importance of historical factors, but referred only infrequently to any events before 1960 and focused mainly on the 1980s. Most of the countries considered in these studies, however, had achieved their distinctive positions in life expectancy before the 1960s. The key period was not 1960 to 1990, but 1890 to 1960, especially 1920 to 1960.

My goal in this book is to explain the period of achievement, 1890 to 1960, rather than the era of maintenance, since 1960, and to interpret from the historical record. The cast of countries differs, too. Here also Sri Lanka and Costa Rica appear, along with Cuba, and South Korea. Otherwise there is little overlap. China and the Soviet Union will be considered as contrasting versions of a communist model. Japan, Panama, and Jamaica will be included; Mexico will be compared to some other countries in its region. Eight oil-rich lands—Iran, Iraq, Kuwait, Oman, and Saudi Arabia in the Middle East, Algeria and Libya in North Africa, and Venezuela—complete the group, although only Venezuela and Oman receive sustained attention. The twelve extended case studies provided below include countries that attained high life expectancies by 1960 but later fell back, countries that began as both poor and low-survival lands but became rich and high-survival, and countries with extraordinary resources in oil. They also include the classic cases of countries that elevated life expectancy at birth to more than 70 years without ever breaking out of their position as low-income lands. This wide group of case studies provides another test of the different explanations that have been suggested and another opportunity to find explanations for why some countries stand out.

The fundamental questions remain these: How did these countries manage to match the rich lands in life expectancy? What can be learned from their historical experience? Does their experience expose policies that might be followed today and in the future by low-income lands that have not yet achieved high life expectancy, even those countries with a heavy burden of HIV/AIDS? And does their experience shed light on options available to the rich lands that already have high life expectancy but also have health systems that are too costly?

In addition to the different time focus, the main argument here differs as well, for in this research social justice, primary health care, and effective political leadership play secondary roles. What matters most, this study suggests, is that people come to understand disease risks and how to manage them.

Economic Growth and Social Growth

Britain and Belgium initiated modern economic growth in the period 1780–1820 by adding textile-producing factories to their existing handicraft systems of manufacturing and to already well-developed sectors of agriculture and of local and international trade. The term *modern economic growth* refers to industrial modernization, initially in textiles, but from the 1840s also in chemicals, iron and steel, food processing, and other areas, which laid the foundations for sustained economic growth. Economic growth generally preceded and led rising life expectancy in the countries that began health transitions the earliest. The first group, the pioneers, included not only Britain and Belgium but also France, the Nordic lands, and Canada. In the second generation of countries were Germany, the

Netherlands, Italy, the United States, Australia, and New Zealand. Those countries initiated sustained economic growth at different points within the period 1770 to 1900, and in the same period they began to differentiate themselves from other parts of the world by making life expectancy gains.[6]

Thus, when Thomas McKeown looked for a feature of British experience that could be generalized to much of the rest of the world to explain improving survival and the population growth that accompanied it, he found that feature in the idea of a rising standard of living, not in the early decades of industrialization but in the later decades, when wages and many of the amenities of life were undoubtedly improving even for people who worked in factories.[7] McKeown argued that economic modernization played a central role in the health transition, and that populations and societies needed to develop their political, legal, and economic institutions in certain ways as a foundation for other kinds of change. Scholars continue to debate McKeown's ancillary claim that better nutrition constituted the most important territory in which the standard of living improved, but most accept the idea that economic modernization led to improvements in health in these Western countries.

This pattern of sustained economic growth with improved health and longevity proved to be difficult for other countries around the world to copy. Only a few countries, such as Japan and, much more irregularly, the Soviet Union, managed to begin and persist in economic growth within the period 1900–1960, while in others brief periods of growth could not be kept going long enough to achieve high-income status. Most of the world remained economically undeveloped up to the middle of the twentieth century amid circumstances in which the possibility of initiating sustained growth seemed as often to recede as to come within a low-income country's grasp.

Nonetheless, except for Oman, all twelve countries considered at length in this book began to make sustained gains in population survival within the period 1890 to 1940. (Omani citizens began sustained improvements in life expectancy at some point between the 1940s and 1970s.) At the various beginning points of those gains, none of these countries was as impoverished as the lowest-income countries of the late twentieth century. All had attained a certain degree of economic development; they were tied into international trade and finance; and they had at least minimal resources for their inhabitants and their governments to invest in things other than subsistence. Although the people in these countries and their leaders hoped for sustained economic growth and tried to promote it, many of them failed, remaining low-income lands. These countries fared better, however, at building the institutions, habits of mind, and behaviors of social growth.

Social development and social growth require some specification. One approach to this issue takes the experience of European and other Western countries as a model and seeks to understand their social growth. The most comprehensive investigation of the development of government spending on social transfers, which is the way most Western countries have engaged in social development, shows that, hesitantly from the 1880s and then more aggressively from the 1930s and 1940s, Western governments spent rising shares of their budgets and rising proportions of national income on public health, education, poor relief and family assistance, unemployment compensation, publicly funded pensions, and housing subsidies. The countries in western Europe plus Australia, Canada, New Zealand, and the United States were able to make such investments because they were already far along in economic development. But they were actually led to make such investments, Peter Lindert argues, because they had open and democratic political regimes, aging populations, and values associated with Protestantism.[8]

Scholars interested in the problem of development in low-income countries and the uneven stages and paces of development among countries have sometimes described social growth as an alternative path to economic growth via industrialization. Arthur Livingstone wrote about the elements of social growth in 1969 in a short book treating education, health, social welfare, the determinants of social policy, and the instruments of social policy in the third world. His aim was to foster the development of these factors as ways to escape poverty and hunger. Livingstone recognized the importance of many specific elements of social growth, including adult education, the education of women, teacher training, health education, access to health services for the rural population, and health care for mothers, infants, and children. But he did not imagine that many countries had already made remarkable progress in developing the institutions of social growth and finding resources to sustain them, believing instead that countries marred by poverty and underdevelopment showed a "curious ambivalence" toward education, uneven progress in disease control, and uncertainty about which elements of social welfare to try to promote.[9] Of course, many did. But the important point is that some did not, that some low-income lands had already made substantial progress in developing social institutions.

As noted above, five areas of social growth claim special attention here because they are the central areas of action through which the low-income lands under study managed to elevate life expectancy. These countries made small but persistent investments in public health, education, and health care, in people's understanding of health risks, and in people's participation in improving their own survival prospects. The small investments accumulated. Although they had not set out a plan of social growth in advance, their actions defined such growth. Their investments were in some part financial, usually taking the form of higher spending by central and local government. But these investments came also in ideas and in community organizations and engagement. To existing ideas about family life and survival were added new ideas about how people might improve the circumstances of their lives and more especially the lives of their children. To existing community organizations and leaders—churches and spiritual leaders, healers and midwives, and other people commanding respect—were added new organizations and leaders, such as primary schools and their teachers; local public health programs and their nurses and health inspectors; and clinics and the medical auxiliaries who staffed them.

Ideas about the forms of social growth came mostly from the outside world. The formation of a preference for social growth came from within.

A Theory about Rising Life Expectancy

High life expectancy is the product not of single factors operating with singular strength, but of an accumulating variety of factors that changes over time. Three examples will illustrate this point.

First, beginning in the late nineteenth and early twentieth century, Western cities and towns controlled fecal disease by filtering and chlorinating water and building waterborne systems for the collection and disposal of human waste. Most of the rest of the world has lagged behind in making these sanitary improvements because of their extreme costliness. Some countries have used other, less expensive ways to control fecal disease, the chief of which has been the pit latrine introduced in an improved form in the 1920s, but diseases transmitted in human waste remain an important cause of death in some parts of the world in the early years of the twenty-first century. The control of fecal-borne disease began in the middle of the nineteenth century and has, since then, made uneven and limited progress, pushing forward in different regions of the globe by different means in different periods.

Second, in the period 1945–70 antibiotics are believed to have played a leading role in the treatment of bacterial diseases in developing countries. Antibiotics came too late to have played a leading role in suppressing bacterial disease in the now high-income countries, however, and were too late also in certain low-income lands. Those countries controlled tuberculosis, typhoid fever, and many other bacterial diseases by other means, some of which will be explored below.

Third, many countries used smallpox vaccination sporadically during the nineteenth century, and some of them reduced mortality from smallpox to a low level. But it was the 1970s and 1980s before vaccinations against smallpox and other childhood diseases were widely employed in developing countries, even though many vaccines had been available for some time. Although the same basic technique was used from the introduction of a vaccine in 1796 up to the eradication of this disease in 1978, smallpox control moved forward quite unevenly from place to place and time to time for reasons quite separate from the technology of vaccination itself.

These three examples illustrate the ever-changing supply and deployment of programs and actions that have reduced mortality. In compiling a synthetic portrait of this process in a book titled *Rising Life Expectancy: A Global History,* I divided contributory factors into six categories or tactical areas: public health; medicine; wealth, income, and economic development; famine, malnutrition, and diet; household and individual behavior; and literacy and education. Each encompasses many programs and actions that have proved, at one time and place or another, helpful in elevating survival. The premise of this approach to a theory of rising life expectancy is that different countries and different populations have used different combinations of these many programs and actions. Just as there have been many paths to social development, there have been many paths to high life expectancy.

This premise leads in a different direction from the usual comparative studies of social or economic growth, which attempt to find a leading or dominant explanation that might then serve as the marker for countries that lag. It leads instead to the idea that countries and peoples can select among many options and opportunities, perhaps to find the programs and actions that are most easily adopted in the circumstances that prevail in their country. This approach therefore shifts the emphasis away from proposing substantial reorientations in individual behavior and public policy and toward finding the adaptations that can most readily be made given existing patterns of behavior, habits of mind, institutions, resources, and other characteristics of a country and its people.

Research into how higher rates of survival have been achieved regularly shows that three of the five areas of social growth identified have played a role. Certainly, education has contributed. People with more years of schooling have long enjoyed better health themselves, and mothers with more schooling have raised infants and children with notably higher survival prospects. So has public health, which refers to the provision of safe water and safe ways for disposing of human waste and to many other actions that seek to improve community health. And so has medicine. Scholars continue to debate the value of medicine, but the general public has long believed that consulting a physician or a medical auxiliary is the best way to deal with a sickness that has not resolved itself and that has resisted self-treatment.[10] Scholarly writing about social growth and the attainment of higher life expectancy much less often assigns importance to the other factors: people's understanding of the health risks they face and how to temper those risks, or their participation in the effort to improve their own lives and survival prospects. This book presents extensive evidence of popular participation and of the engagement of individuals and households in social growth and in managing health risks. It shows that reliance on the capacity of ordinary people to learn how to improve their own position played a role not just in individualistic and capitalist societies, such as Jamaica, but also in the Soviet Union and China.

Fecal Disease, Malaria, and Tuberculosis

Individuals die, in most instances, for reasons related, firstly, to a specific disease or injury or two or more co-morbidities and, secondly, to the circumstances of their lives: poverty, housing, access to health care, education, occupation, diet, prior wellness or sickness, among many other factors. Populations, too, confront disease and injury as well as these background factors, which may determine whether people are exposed to disease, whether they fall sick, how severe an episode will be, and whether there are significant co-morbidities.

Certain diseases played a leading part as causes of death in the period 1890–1940, when most of the countries to be considered here began to make sustained gains in survival. Three important diseases were malaria; pulmonary tuberculosis; and the complex of diseases that includes dysentery, typhoid fever, and unspecified diarrheas that share the characteristic of being communicated in human fecal matter. Fecal disease, malaria, and tuberculosis killed some people at every age, but they had their most profound impact on infants, children, youths, and young adults, up to age 30 or so. Because these diseases accounted for such a large share of deaths, it was extraordinarily difficult for any country to make sustained progress in survival without reducing mortality from at least two of the three. Malaria and a heavy burden of certain parasites communicated through fecal matter, including hookworm, also played the part of co-morbidities: they were debilitating diseases that added to the likelihood that someone would fall sick from another cause and perhaps die.

It is worth noting that even today these same diseases continue to play a significant role as causes of death in countries where survival rates are low; modern medicine has not yet managed to suppress them.[11]

In most of the countries to be considered here, the circumstances of people's lives at the beginning point of these country studies, in the 1890s, compounded the risks that people faced. Nearly everyone was poor, compared to elites in their own lands or to the general population in Western Europe and the United States. People lived mostly in houses that were crowded and poorly constructed, with dirt floors, neither running water nor toilets, and with primitive facilities for preserving and cooking food. They ate foods selected from what they could grow, what was available, and what they could afford rather than what would later be determined to be diets balanced in food elements, vitamins, and minerals. They rarely called doctors when they were sick. Either they did not attend school, or the schools they attended instructed them in matters that did little or nothing to enhance their understanding of health risks or their access to information about health. They held certain beliefs about the sources of sickness, but those beliefs were of limited utility for preventing or avoiding disease. These people raised their children according to rules and customs that, likewise, did little to enhance a child's prospects of survival or of remaining well. Even in the most advanced lands, infant mortality did not begin to decline until the late nineteenth century.[12]

The people in low-income countries in the 1890s could not be called docile, but neither were they prepared to assert themselves in the realm of public health; the idea of demanding public investment in their health needs either had not occurred to them or had not yet been seized. At this time the great majority of people died early, in infancy, childhood, youth, or early adulthood, but most commonly in infancy.

Behind these proximate circumstances of life that influenced disease risks stand more distant circumstances, which likewise conspired against survival. These were countries with weak political institutions; their leaders often made laws that could not be enforced or implemented. Thus innovations that might have improved health, such as the public health offices created in some Latin American and Caribbean countries in the late nineteenth century, remained ineffective. There were few roads and railroads, few cities, few industries, and few ways of amassing the resources required to build roads, enlarge cities, or manufacture the goods that people wanted. These countries had small elites and large numbers of poor and powerless people, but little or nothing in the way of a middle class. They had few secular schools or teachers and little capacity to train teachers. They had few hospitals and clinics, and not much in the way of a public health apparatus.

These countries had not yet benefited from the processes of building individual and community wealth already set in motion in the lands then becoming rich. The poor countries thus accumulated much less in physical or human capital than the countries growing rich could do, and the individuals in them seldom managed to hand much down to their children in either a family or a community inheritance, in knowledge useful for economic improvement or for protecting against health hazards.

Four Background Factors

In the years 1890 to 1960, the period of focus in this study, certain conditions began to change in many poor countries. Four background factors in particular influenced survival: urbanization; income distribution; social investments, especially schooling; and the theory and practice of disease management, avoidance, and prevention. All four appear in the case studies that make up the central part of this book, and so a brief review is useful here.

A rising proportion of people living in cities—urbanization—had long been an unrelievedly negative factor in European experience. Death rates in cities surpassed those in rural areas. and that was probably true for non-Western cities as well in the nineteenth century. At different points between about 1890 and 1970, earlier in the rich lands and later in low-income countries, the added risk associated with living in a city gave way to a reduced risk; the urban penalty metamorphosed into a rural penalty. In rich lands urban authorities mastered many of the risks of city life by building systems to deliver safe water and remove human waste.[13] That did not happen in cities in low-income countries, except in elite neighborhoods. But in low-income countries health facilities and resources were ultimately concentrated in cities, giving urban residents much better access than their rural counterparts to whatever advantages medicine could provide. People living in cities also got schools earlier, as well as higher incomes, jobs that allowed them to organize labor unions, and some other advantages. Thus, in the case studies below, urbanization will appear sometimes as a negative and sometimes as a positive factor in population survival, depending on circumstances in a particular country and the period being discussed.

The second thing that changed is that income distribution came to be associated with health. In Europe in the mid-seventeenth century people with higher incomes were unable to use their income or wealth to provide themselves with better protection against health risks. By 1900, however, Europeans with higher incomes had learned how to secure longer survival, so that a marked socio-economic gradient in health had developed in the West. There are signs that income differentiation showing up in health had begun in England in the eighteenth century, but this became much more obvious in the first half of the nineteenth century, in the early stages of industrialization. Indeed, many historians argue that the standard of living of the people then working in textile factories deteriorated, compared to the hypothetical alternative of traditional employments, residences, incomes, and opportunities for leisure.[14] Certainly the lives and livelihoods of urban workers exposed them to survival hazards much greater than those faced by urban elites or, indeed, rural agriculturalists.

Europeans living in colonies in Asia and the Americas acquired the advantages of high-income groups in the metropole during the nineteenth century. So did soldiers; the risk that a European soldier serving in the British Caribbean, Algeria, tropical and southern Africa, or India would die was by 1900 dramatically less than it had been in the 1830s.[15] There is not yet enough evidence to say whether risks within indigenous populations in these colonies and elsewhere were distributed by income by 1900. They certainly were by 1950. Thus outside the West, too, a greater skew in the distribution of income led eventually to a health-and-income hierarchy, in which people with the lowest incomes had far more abridged chances of survival.

Income distribution will come up several times in the case studies assembled here, making it useful to start with some sense of the proportion and trend of changes in distribution. Sweden is a useful example because it has been studied intensively and because Swedes ultimately decided to favor an atypically egalitarian distribution.[16] Up to the 1950s the best estimates for Sweden rely on the differential in wages paid skilled and unskilled laborers. Those indicate that inequality rose in the period from 1750 to 1914, then briefly leveled off. The differential increased again into the early 1930s, then decreased from the 1930s to the 1950s.[17] Figure 1 provides estimates of the inequality in distribution of family or household income from 1951 to 1996 in three curves, one showing the distribution before and the other two after transfer payments, such as pensions to retired people, which promote greater equality. Swedes decided in the years after World War II to use government transfer payments to equalize income distribution, and this figure shows that they succeeded. However, in Sweden periods of improving life expectancy since 1750 have not usually coincided with periods of movement toward a more egalitarian income distribution. Thus Sweden's experience does not support the argument that uneven distributions, at least in middle- and high-income countries, impede survival. Nor do international comparisons in general support this idea.[18]

In another way, too, the issue of income distribution poses a thorny problem for this study. What is typically measured is the distribution of income before such transfer payments as pensions and welfare assistance, and without regard for any assistance from family, friends, and church or for benefits obtained from publicly funded activities, such as schools, public health amenities, and clinics. Transfer payments do not pose a big problem for this study because most the countries considered here could not afford to build social security systems, at least not until well into the history of their life expectancy gains. But these countries did make social investments, building a social infrastructure that amounted to a kind of transfer payment to ordinary people who used the schools, public health institutions, clinics, and other resources in the social infrastructure. Because income distribution estimates usually fail to capture such benefits and do not distinguish countries that spend more on social infrastructure, they have limited usefulness for studying differences in the resources available to households.

The third category of change is these investments in social infrastructure, especially in schools, public health improvements, hospitals, institutions to train health providers, clinics, and other health programs and facilities. In many of the low-income countries treated here the scale of investment in such institutions and facilities began to rise before the end of the nineteenth century. The size of social investments can be reconstructed, and such quantitative markers as school enrollments, hospital beds, and the numbers of trained nurses and doctors can often be recovered. But it is virtually impossible to say just how much use people in different income groups made of these investments.

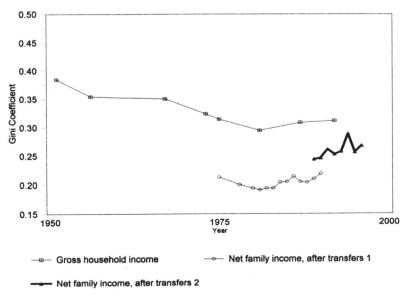

FIGURE I. Inequality in distribution of household income in Sweden, 1951–96, by Gini coefficient. The two curves for transfers represent different packages of transfer payments for those periods.
SOURCES: Anders Björklund and Mårten Palme, "The Evolution of Income Inequality during the Rise of the Swedish Welfare State 1951 to 1973," *Nordic Journal of Political Economy* 26 (2000): 115–28; and the United Nations Development Programme, World Income Inequality Database at http://www.wider.unu.edu/wiid/wwwwiid.htm, accessed March 24, 2005.

Nineteenth-century Europeans came to see schools as pathways to a better life for the succeeding generation, and that hopeful view spread into many European colonies and to independent lands toward the end of the nineteenth century and afterwards. Modern research shows that schooling and literacy transform the sources of information available to people, instill greater confidence, and, when girls are schooled, give women a basis from which to negotiate more effectively with male partners. In Western countries the period 1870–1920 was apparently an era of transition from circumstances in which schooling conveyed little survival advantage to an individual or a community to circumstances in which it would ordinarily convey a sizeable advantage.[19]

The schools were also a platform for teaching health lessons. In the period 1870–1920 primary schools commonly added lessons in hygiene and taught children how to avoid particular diseases. In many countries schools were the principal avenue for instructing people in practical lessons about how diseases are transmitted. Thus building primary schools, training teachers, and enrolling children in school transformed the possibilities that countries had for improving health, even though that was nowhere the reason that schools were built. In most of the world around 1850 schooling and literacy were not things that individuals valued, for themselves or their children. By 1960 quite the reverse was true.

The fourth area of change covers two bodies of theory developed in the nineteenth-century West, each seeking to explain the origins of disease and, therefore, how to avoid, prevent, or manage disease. The main body of theory available in 1870 was filth theory, which held that epidemic diseases arise from uncleanliness, from matter giving off offensive odors, or from the odors themselves, and that diseases are transmitted through the air or in water. Filth theory led to the idea that the human habitat should be cleaned up, that people should avoid contact with human waste, that water should be filtered or drawn from sources not contaminated with filth, that housing should be airy, and, by this date, that people should wash face and hands every day and bathe often, at least once a week. The germ theory of disease as it developed in the 1870s and 1880s acted to reinforce the prescriptions for cleanliness in filth theory, albeit for different reasons.

For present purposes what matters most about both theories is that each could provide information necessary to formulate simple advice that ordinary people could deploy to avoid disease. By the 1890s commentators were extracting such principles, and they were using the schools, pamphlets and books, lectures, and illustrations (many devised to reach people who could not read) to instruct the public in health lessons. Changes in this area came in two forms, one dealing with the content of filth and germ theory and the other with the selection of practical advice that ordinary people might adopt. The low-income countries that began early health transitions drew on Western ideas about disease causation and transmission, on Western models of health education, and on the comparatively new Western practice of using public resources to try to improve population health.

Against the background of these four changes, we now turn to the changing relationship between life expectancy and income.

CHAPTER I

Life Expectancy and Income among the First Countries to Begin Health Transitions

Life Expectancy

Within the last two centuries every country around the globe has experienced sustained periods of progress in survival, with health transitions beginning as early as the 1770s and as recently as the 1970s.[1] Around 1800, when some countries were beginning their transitions, life expectancy at birth was as low as 22.5 years in the indigenous populations of Oceania and as high as 34.8 years in some parts of the Americas. The global average was about 28.5 years. (Life expectancy at birth measures the current probability of surviving at each age for the year in question, rather than the actual survival prospects of a person born that year. Thus it gives the best assessment available of population survival that year.)

Working with countries of the world as they were identified in 2000 rather than with the much more ambiguous boundaries and identities of 1800, and considering survival in the decades just before each country began its health transition, the lowest pre-transition life expectancy was perhaps 20.1 years (Pakistan) and the highest 40 to 42 years (Scotland, Switzerland, the United States).[2] The overall average across countries in the periods when they began health transitions was 33.1 years.[3] Both that and the 1800 average were higher than the life expectancy of 20–25 years at the transition from Paleolithic to Neolithic populations, around the domestication of plants and animals, but only by a few years.[4] Thus, a true revolution in survival has occurred since 1800, with most of the gains having come since 1920.

Such estimates of life expectancy average across long periods for pre-

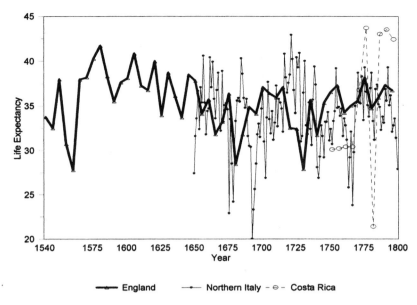

FIGURE 2. Life expectancy in England, northern Italy and Costa Rica, 1540–1800. (Wars, epidemics, and famines all may cause sudden and severe declines in survival.)
SOURCES: Patrick R. Galloway, "A Reconstruction of the Population of North Italy from 1650 to 1881 Using Annual Inverse Projection with Comparison to England, France and Sweden," *European Journal of Population* 10 (1994): 223–74; Héctor Pérez Brignoli, *El crecimiento demográfico de America Latina en los siglos XIX y XX: Problemas, metodos y perspectives* (San José: Centro de Investigaciones Historicas, Universidad de Costa Rica, 1989), p. 12; and E. A. Wrigley and R. S. Schofield, *The Population History of England, 1541–1871: A Reconstruction* (Cambridge: Cambridge University Press, 1989), pp. 528–29.

transition levels, going back as far, in the case of England, as the 1540s and, for northern Italy, the 1650s. Although early year-to-year and period-to-period estimates for three regions (England, northern Italy and Costa Rica; figure 2) do show waves of rising and falling survival prospects, there was still no strong indication of a long-run trend in that early period.

Nonetheless, some countries had made significant gains in survival, and by 1800 the world was divided between higher and lower survival regions. The countries in northwestern Europe, from the United Kingdom to Norway, Sweden, and Iceland, belonged to a high survival region, as did also Japan and Costa Rica. But France, British India, and the slave populations of the British Caribbean faced lower survival prospects.[5] It is not yet possible to say much about when or under what circumstances the early shifts toward higher survival occurred. And it remains possible that some of the higher survival areas had enjoyed that status back to Paleolithic times.

For the moment the most important inference to be drawn is that life expectancy was variable but not trended in the pre-transition era, varying usually within the range from 25 to 35 years.[6] There is no indication of progressively improving human management of mortality risks, although there are many ways in which humans in 1800 were better at controlling the disease and injury risks in their environment than their counterparts had been around the time of the Neolithic Revolution. The problem was that many of the things people did in building their civilizations also aggravated those risks. On the positive side, societies across the world collected knowledge about herbal treatments for disease and injury, and educated a body of health care providers in the accumulated and collective wisdom of their cultures about how to prevent and treat disease and injury. Some of the concoctions they used and some of the things they knew appear, in retrospect, to have been useful, though others seem to have been largely beside the point and some even harmful. Also, in some countries people deferred marriage and thereby reduced fertility along with infant and child mortality.

On the negative side, most human communities traded with their neighbors, allowed people to move from place to place, and formed urban concentrations of population, all of which had adverse effects. Trade and migration carried communicable diseases from place to place and contributed to a microbial unification of the globe in which people would be exposed to unfamiliar diseases brought from afar. Towns and cities meant that people lived closer together, transmitting airborne diseases more efficiently. The provisions they had made for the disposal of human waste and refuse in sparsely settled rural areas were not sufficient to protect them from disease in the urban setting. Many towns or cities sought to control disease, but few had found anything approaching effective measures, judged in the light of today's understanding of disease transmission. The net effect was higher mortality in towns and cities than in rural areas. For example, Stockholm's life expectation in the 1890s, 43.0 years, was about ten years less than the expectation in rural areas.[7] In general in the same period rural farm laborers, who did not own land and worked irregularly, lived longer than any occupational group living in cities.

Only a few countries managed to initiate health transitions before the 1870s. One of these can be used to illustrate the longer history of survivorship. Figure 3 shows the reconstructed life expectancy history of, suc-

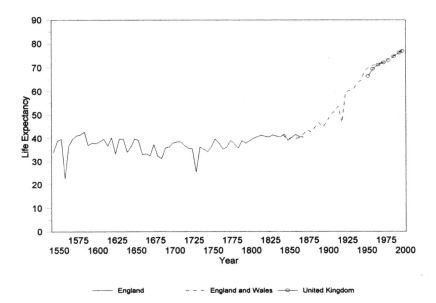

FIGURE 3. Life expectancy in England, England and Wales, and the United Kingdom, 1540s to 2000.
SOURCES: (England) E. A. Wrigley et al., *English Population History from Family Reconstitution, 1580–1837* (Cambridge: Cambridge University Press, 1997), pp. 614–15 (E. A. Wrigley and R. S. Schofield, *The Population History of England, 1541–1871: A Reconstruction* [Cambridge: Cambridge University Press, 1989], pp. 528–29, indicate similar levels and a similar path of life expectancy for England in the overlapping period); (England and Wales) Human Mortality Database, www.mortality.org, accessed various dates in 2004; (United Kingdom) World Bank, *World Development Indicators 2004 on CD-ROM* (Washington: World Bank, 2004).

cessively, England, England and Wales, and the United Kingdom from the 1540s to 2000. Gains in survival began in the first decade of the nineteenth century, but were meager until the period 1900–1950. The urban penalty persisted in England until the last years of the nineteenth century. During the nineteenth century it slowed the pace of life expectancy gains even though survival prospects were improving in both cities and rural areas, taken separately. But the main point made with figure 3 is the deliberate pace of progress among the pioneers. They began early, and they all achieved high life expectancy, but for the most part they moved toward a life expectancy at birth above 75 years much more slowly than would be the case for countries that began health transitions later.

Gains in Material Prosperity

In the material circumstances of life, in contrast, many human communities had by 1800 made noteworthy progress since the ancient domestication of plants and animals, and some had made substantial progress. While this is easy enough to assert with confidence, it is more difficult to suggest values for the level of material comfort or the standard of living. The standard of comparison used today is most often the gross domestic product per capita (GDPpc) expressed in values adjusted for price change.

Two important factors, however, wealth and the things that people produce for themselves, are rarely considered as part of GDP. First, the accumulated stock the community has in housing; improvements to infrastructure, such as roads, ships, farms, and workshops; human learning; and all the other things that constitute resources for growth, must of course be counted as wealth rather than as product. It is usually quite difficult to gauge the sum of this accumulated wealth for a single country, much less to make comparisons among countries or across time. If the main goal is to estimate economic growth, then GDP and each year's addition to GDP may give a rough idea about the scale of wealth. That is, like the interest on a treasury note, the annual yield gives a way to estimate the size of the capital behind that yield. But the goal here is to understand gains in survival, which are related to a society's wealth but not directly products of it. For both the level of life expectancy and the prospect of improving it, some forms of wealth are more important than others, and returns on wealth do not adequately capture the difference. This can be illustrated by an aside dealing with smallpox vaccination.

Smallpox was the leading cause of death in northwestern Europe in the eighteenth century and probably a leading cause of death in most global regions in the same period. In regions where the disease was endemic, children around age 1 were most susceptible. Where smallpox was unfamiliar, people of all ages were susceptible. Edward Jenner introduced vaccination against smallpox in England in 1796 and not long thereafter speculated that this technique could make it possible to eradicate smallpox everywhere.

Vaccination was first used effectively, as a mass population technique to reduce mortality, in the Nordic lands in the early years of the nineteenth century. Those countries had quite significantly lower income levels than England or than most other countries neighboring England, but they were better prepared to take advantage of smallpox vaccination. What mattered, as Peter Sköld has shown, was not just the invention of vaccination but also the capacity to deploy it widely enough to curtail smallpox mortality. Sweden moved to control smallpox faster and earlier than most other countries in Europe by "constructing a system of health related laws" and deploying leadership from the center via an effective administrative system that was able to assemble a large enough number of vaccinators, most of them neither medical practitioners nor government officials and including many members of the clergy. The Swedish people accepted vaccination much more readily than they had accepted the earlier practice of inoculation, which tried to protect against the dangers of smallpox by inducing a mild case. In contrast, vaccination protected by using the much less dangerous cowpox material to deceive the immune system into building antibodies against smallpox. In Sweden a compulsory vaccination law was adopted in 1816, with a fine to punish parents who did not get their children vaccinated. Mortality from smallpox had already dropped sharply from 1810, however, showing that it was not compulsion but other characteristics of Sweden's vaccination program that mattered the most. Other countries adopted laws compelling vaccination but did not succeed in getting such a large share of the population vaccinated so quickly and often did not succeed in enforcing their laws on compulsory vaccination.[8]

The institutions that made vaccination an early success in Sweden existed ahead of time, rather than being created for the moment. The two novelties were vaccination itself and its general acceptance by the people. That acceptance was, in Sköld's telling of this history, a product of the successful outcome of early practice with vaccination, from 1802. People were prepared to adopt a new public health practice where it was shown to be successful and where community leaders supported it. Continued acceptance was assisted also by the government's openness in publishing statistics about vaccinations and the successful outcome of the early vaccinations.

The history of smallpox vaccination in Sweden suggests that social organization and social habits, trustworthy leadership, and openness in communicating information mattered more than per capita income and economic resources in determining whether children would be protected against smallpox. Thus the important point is that Sweden's social organization was well suited to the conquest of smallpox, but not so well suited to generating a high level of, or large annual gains in, GDP. Social organization constitutes a form of wealth that played the key role in protecting Swedish children against smallpox, but is not an asset of the type that is ordinarily counted as wealth.

The second group of items that GDP estimates typically exclude are the things people produce for themselves that do not pass through markets. The food people grow for themselves; the houses they build and improve; the learning that occurs outside of formal schooling, such as acquiring the skills associated with farming or with a trade, and learning from parents; the services provided within a household or between households without any exchange of cash; and many other products, services, and behaviors therefore go unmeasured. New information may also be a form of income when it enhances the standard of living. Learning about how to avoid or manage a disease may, like learning a skill, add to well-being. These unmeasured goods differ in scale from time to time and from country to country, so that making comparisons across time and space is difficult. Yet the differences are hugely important for comparisons across broad swaths of time and for comparing poor and rich countries at the same dates.

Phyllis Deane developed the approach usually taken in trying to account for transactions outside the cash economy in a study of social accounting in colonial Nyasaland and Northern Rhodesia in the early 1950s. Her case study draws attention to the disparities between the cash economy, in which the Europeans living there operated most of the time, and the non-cash economy, where Africans operated much of the time in "inter-village trade" and "goods and services produced for home consumption." That parallel made it easy enough to discover the cash value of many products and services exchanged in the non-cash economy, so that Deane was able to give a plausible estimate of the 1945 subsistence and barter incomes of Africans in Northern Rhodesia. According to her estimate, the Africans' subsistence and barter activity nearly matched their cash incomes. But Deane did not try to measure all types of activity in the informal economy, omitting, among other items, illegal activity and the labor of dependents within a household, and she did not draw a contrast between the accumulated wealth of most Europeans, which made it easier for them to generate incomes, and that of Africans, which was meager and less productive of income or survival. It was clear enough that Europeans were much better off than Africans: Deane estimated European income at about £600 per earner versus about £27 per adult male African.[9]

It is more difficult to produce plausible estimates of income for people living in subsistence economies without parallel cash economies, as is true for most historical communities and for the informal sectors of modern economies. The term *informal economy* describes the parts of an economy in which transactions are hidden, whether because they occur by barter, in illegal or quasi-legal activity, or in unreported cash transactions. In the informal economy people deliberately obfuscate income and consumption in order to avoid taxation, conceal illegal activities, or obtain eligibility for social services for which they would not otherwise qualify. Rough estimates of the size of the informal economy in Jamaica place it at 39 percent of formal economy activity in 1989.[10] Janet MacGaffey argues that actual economic activity around 1990 in Zaire (Democratic Republic of the Congo) may have been three times greater than the official GDP, amidst rapid growth in the informal sector.[11] Thus the unobserved part of income may be quite substantial, and it may be significant even in a developed economy. Estimates of the scale of black market activity in England in the 1970s range from a low of 2 to a high of 15 percent, but were probably closer to the lower figure.[12]

Scholars who have tried to assess levels of output broadly across time and space have sometimes adopted a simplifying device, which is to assign a minimum level of GDPpc to poor and primitive economies. Angus Maddison appears to have had such a device in mind in assigning the value of 400 international (or purchasing power parity) dollars of 1990 to GDPpc in Australia for 1500–1700 and New Zealand for 1500–1840, before the arrival of Europeans and in a period when there was no cash economy. But Maddison later deviates from this approach by assigning lower values to a number of countries in Africa for various parts of the period 1950–2001, including Botswana in the 1950s and Chad in the 1980s. For Zaire in 2001 he estimates GDPpc at only 202 international dollars of 1990. Thus Maddison suggests that per capita income in the Maori population of New Zealand in 1800 was about twice as high as it was in Zaire in 2001.[13] Presumably he means to estimate output as money transactions in the formal economy, excluding smuggling, an important activity in Congo in 2001, and many other things that added to the material standard of living there. (Since so many of the amounts that will be referenced below will be given in international dollars of 1990, it is convenient to adopt an abbreviation of I$. Unless otherwise indicated, in this book the symbol I$ always refers to 1990 values. Using U.S. experience with price change as a rough guide, I$ 100 in 1990 was equal to about I$ 150 in 2005.)[14]

What is implied by the I$ 400 floor (or any other floor) is that people living within the market sector could supply themselves with their basic needs for that sum. In truth the sum of I$ 400 is much too low a value to assign to the output of the average person living in a primitive economy in the past or a low-income country in the modern world. The idea behind this number is that, on average, the people in a primitive or poor community live at a subsistence level, just meeting their basic needs in food, housing, fuel and heat, apparel, and so forth. But it is difficult to imagine how those needs could be met with a money equivalent of I\$ 400. What level should be preferred is little more than guesswork, but may be as much as several times higher. It is not possible actually to correct Maddison's estimates to incorporate economic activity outside the formal and cash sectors because scaling up the floor of GDPpc estimates also involves scaling up all lower-range estimates.

Since many low-income countries have a larger share of economic activity outside the cash and formal economies than do most high-income countries, underestimation of income from these activities will understate actual levels of GDPpc in low-income countries more than in high-income countries. Thus Maddison's approach tends, by understating income in poor countries, to exaggerate the difference between poor and rich countries.

The GDPpc approach also tends to overstate income in rich lands by counting all forms of economic activity on the same footing. The rich lands produce many items that are far removed from food, housing, clothing, and other necessities for survival, and those items, such as a second house and a car for each adult, add to income levels. In a way, then, the rich lands appear to be better off than they actually are, judged by the standards that prevail in poor lands. Since the outcome in judging economic growth is the sum of GDP, any activity that generates income appears to have equivalent merit, per unit of income. GDPpc estimates therefore mask elements of income in rich lands that are more superficial than substantial. Nonetheless, although both factors—economic activity in the informal or invisible sector and the practice of counting all visible economic activity on the same footing—tend to exaggerate the difference in actual income levels between rich and poor lands, there is no question but that the low-income lands are poor.

Despite these important shortcomings in measuring and comparing income, it is useful to consider how far differences in life expectancy may be related to differences in national income. As the next section will show, most of this consideration can rely at least initially on Western countries, for which estimates of GDP back to 1820 or even earlier have a much stronger foundation than do the estimates made for other parts of the world in the eighteenth and nineteenth century.

Life Expectancy and Income: An Evolving Relationship

Maddison estimates GDPpc values across the globe in 1820 for thirty-eight countries in I\$. (Again, all I\$ values continue to be given in terms of con-

TABLE 1. Gross Domestic Product per Capita (GDPpc) in 1990 International Dollars (I$) and Life Expectancy circa 1820 in 14 Countries

	GDPpc (1990 I$)	Life Expectancy
Belgium	1,319	32.3 years
Canada	904	39.0
China	600	35.5
Denmark	1,274	44.4
England, Wales, and Scotland	2,121	39.0
Finland	781	37.1
France	1,135	38.2
Germany	1,077	40.3
Greece	641	29.0
Ireland	877	38.3
Italy	1,117	34.9
Norway	1,104	47.8
Spain	1,008	26.8
Sweden	1,198	39.7

SOURCES: *For GDPpc estimates*: Angus Maddison, *The World Economy: Historical Statistics* (Paris: Development Center of the Organization for Economic Cooperation and Development, 2003), pp. 58–59, 87, 100, 142, 146, 180–81; *for England, Wales, and Scotland*: Angus Maddison, *The World Economy: A Millennial Perspective* (Paris: Development Center of the Organization for Economic Cooperation and Development, 2001), p. 247. *For life expectancy estimates: Belgium*, averaging three closely-spaced estimates for 1827, 1829, and 1832, J.-M.-J Leclerc, "Tables de mortalité ou de survie et table de population pour la Belgique, dressées au moyen des statistiques officielles de 1880 à 1890," *Bulletin de la commis-*

stant 1990 dollars.) These show sharp differences in the material standard among these countries, ranging from a low of I$ 400 in New Zealand to a high of I$ 2,121 in England, Wales, and Scotland.[15] Life expectancy estimates are available for fourteen of these thirty-eight countries, and those are given together with Maddison's GDPpc estimates in table 1. This is just enough cases to allow analysis of the statistical association between GDPpc and life expectancy. The result is a very small association (adjusted R-square of −0.003) lacking statistical significance.[16] Among these countries, then, with most of them on the eve or in the early stages of health transitions but after significant periods of economic progress, higher average incomes around 1820 did not coincide with elevated survival prospects.

Thirty-one countries initiated health transitions between the 1770s and the 1890s. Table 2 shows the period when sustained gains began plus the life expectancy level and Maddison's estimates of GDPpc for the twenty-four countries for which both are available at that point. (Appendix 1 gives *sion centrale de statistique* 17 (1890–96): 65, and A. Quetelet, "Nouvelles tables de mortalité pour la Belgique," *Bulletin de la commission centrale de statistique* 4 (1851): 18–19. *Canada,* Robert Bourbeau and Jacques Légaré, *Evolution de la mortalité au Canada et au Québec, 1831–1931: Essai de mesure par génération* (Montreal: Presses de l'Université de Montréal, 1982), their estimate centered on 1831. *China,* the mid-point of the estimate for 1800–1850 from William Lavely and R. Bin Wong, "Revising the Malthusian Narrative: The Comparative Study of Population Dynamics in Late Imperial China," *Journal of Asian Studies* 57 (1998): 714–48. *Denmark,* averaging estimates for 1817 and 1822 from Otto Andersen, "Denmark," in *European Demography and Economic Growth,* ed. W. R. Lee (London: Croom Helm, 1979), p. 111. *England, Wales, and Scotland,* the average of estimates for England for 1816–26 from E. A. Wrigley and R. S. Schofield, *The Population History of England, 1541–1871: A Reconstruction* (Cambridge: Cambridge University Press, 1989), p. 529. *Finland,* averaging estimates for 1815 and 1825 from Väinö Kannisto, Mauri Nieminen, and Oiva Turpeinen, "Finnish Life Tables since 1751," *Demographic Research* 1 (1999), at www.demographic-research.org/ Volumes/Vol1/1. *France,* the average of estimates for each year 1818–22, from France Meslé and Jacques Vallin, "Reconstitution de tables annuelles de mortalité pour la France au XIXe siècle," *Population* 44 (1989): 1121–58. *Germany,* the average of estimates centered on 1810 and 1820 from Arthur E. Imhof, ed., *Lebenserwartungen in Deutschland, Norwegen und Schweden im 19. und 20. Jahrhundert* (Berlin: Akademie Verlag, 1994), p. 464. *Greece,* the estimate for 1850 from George Siampos, *Mortality Decline and Longevity in Greece* [in Greek] (Athens: Anotate Schole Oikonomikon kai Emporikon Epistemon, 1989), p. 416. *Ireland,* the estimate for 1821–41 from Phelim P. Boyle and Cormac Ó Gráda, "Fertility Trends, Excess Mortality, and the Great Irish Famine," *Demography* 23 (1986): 543–62. *Italy,* the average of estimates for North Italy for 1818–22 from Patrick R. Galloway, "A Reconstruction of the Population of North Italy from 1650 to 1881 Using Annual Inverse Projection with Comparison to England, France and Sweden," *European Journal of Population* 10 (1994): 223–74. *Norway,* the average of estimates centered on 1818 and 1823 from Helge Brunborg, "The Inverse Projection Method Applied to Norway, 1735–1974," unpublished typescript, July 1976. *Spain,* the estimate for the second half of the eighteenth century from Fausto Dopico and Robert Rowland, "Demografía del censo de Floridablanca: Una aproximación," *Revista de historia económica* 8 (1990): 591–618. *Sweden,* the average of the estimates for 1818–22 from the Human Mortality Database at www.mortality.org.

a complete schedule for the beginning periods of health transitions in 167 countries, the 166 with 2004 populations of at least 400,000 plus Iceland.) With the exception of Canada, the twenty-eight countries for which GDPpc levels can be estimated were above I$ 1,000 at the initiation of health transitions.[17] And most had significantly higher levels still, with an average of I$ 1,831. In terms of GPDpc in constant dollars, the countries listed in table 2 had a noteworthy advantage over the lowest income and survival countries of the nineteenth century or even of the period 1950–2000, many of which neither attained income levels as high as these nor managed to inaugurate sustained economic growth.

   According to Maddison's GDPpc estimates, a few countries achieved levels above I$ 1,000 but did not begin health transitions until later. All of these countries—Bulgaria, Chile, Greece, Portugal, Romania, Sri Lanka, and Uruguay—initiated health transitions by the 1920s. Among them only Chile, with a 1900 GDPpc of I$ 1,949, and Uruguay with I$

TABLE 2. Life Expectancy and Gross Domestic Product per Capita (GDPpc)
at the Beginning of Health Transitions in 24 Countries

Period When Health Transition Began	Country	Life Expectancy around Initiation of Health Transition	GDPpc around Initiation of Health Transition (1990 international dollars)
1770s	Denmark	c. 33	1,039 in 1700; 1,274 in 1820
1790s	France	28.1	910 in 1700; 1,135 in 1820
	Sweden	35.3	977 in 1700; 1,198 in 1820
1800s	England and Wales	36.3 (England only)	2,006 in 1801
1810s	Norway	38.3	1,104 in 1820
1820s or 1830s	Canada	39.0	904 in 1820
1840s	Belgium	38.3	1,694 in 1846
1820s to 1890s	Ireland	38.3	1,775 in 1870
1860s or 1870s	Australia	48.0	3,273 in 1870
	Netherlands	37.3	2,757 in 1870
	New Zealand	51.8–53.1	3,100 in 1870
1860s to 1900s	Mexico	24–29	1,011 in 1890; 1,366 in 1900
1870s	Finland	32.1	1,211 in 1875
	Germany	36.7–38.4	2,112 in 1875
	Switzerland	40.3–40.7	2,645 in 1875

2,219, seem to be cases where the level of economic development
markedly outran development of the factors capable of supporting survival gains.

Most other countries had lower levels of income in the nineteenth century. A GDPpc of roughly I$ 1,000 would appear to have been a threshold
for initiating gains in survival. But most of these countries reached
higher levels before beginning health transitions. Argentina, the Netherlands, Switzerland, and the United States stand out as countries that
might, if GDPpc mattered particularly in the initiation of survival gains
in the nineteenth century, have begun transitions earlier than they appear to have done.[18]

Figure 4 shows the relationship between GDPpc in 1990 I$ and life

TABLE 2. (*continued*)

Period When Health Transition Began	Country	Life Expectancy around Initiation of Health Transition	GDPpc around Initiation of Health Transition (1990 international dollars)
1870s or 1880s	Italy	35.4	1,581 in 1880
1870s to 1890s	Japan	36.6	1,012 in 1890
	United States	39.4	3,106 in 1885
1880s or 1890s	Austria	31.7	2,443 in 1890
1890s	Czech Republic	35	1,505 in 1890
	Spain	29.5	1,689 in 1895
1890s or 1900s	Argentina	33.3	2,756 in 1900
	Russia	31	1,237 in 1900
1890s to 1920s	Costa Rica	30.5	1,624 in 1920

SOURCES: Angus Maddison, *The World Economy: Historical Statistics* (Paris: Development Center of the Organization for Economic Cooperation and Development, 2003), pp. 58–59, 87, 100, 142, 146, 180–81; Maddison, *The World Economy: A Millennial Perspective* (Paris: Development Center of the Organization for Economic Cooperation and Development, 2001), p. 247; James C. Riley, "Bibliography of Works Providing Estimates of Life Expectancy at Birth and of the Beginning Period of Health Transitions in Countries with a Population in 2000 of at least 400,000" at www.lifetable.de/RileyBib.htm.

expectancy periodically from 1820 to 2001. And table 3 shows results from linear regression analysis of associations between the two factors. Among the countries for which both estimates are available at each comparison date, the relationship between per capita income and life expectancy at birth has evolved over time. For 1820, figure 4(a) shows a cluster without any statistical association. By 1870, in a larger group of countries with more dissimilar histories in income and life expectancy, the association was linear, and by 1913 it was at its most robust. For 1950, 1973, and 2001 the association was curvilinear, with or without the outliers, which are oil-rich states (Kuwait in 1950, and Kuwait, Qatar, and the United Arab Emirates in 1973). Judging by the adjusted R-square value, the linear association developed between 1820 and 1870 among the mostly Western countries represented by the analysis.[19] That association reached a peak around 1913 and then weakened.[20]

FIGURE 4 (a–f). Gross domestic product per capita (GDPpc) in 1990 international dollars (I\$) and life expectancy, in 1820, 1870, 1913, 1950, 1973, and 2001. (Please take note of changes in the horizontal axis across time.)

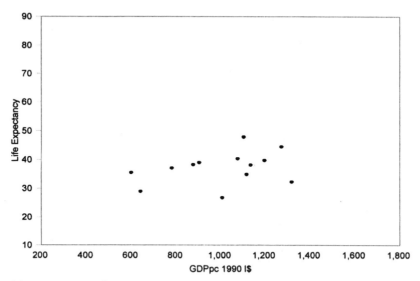

(a) 1820: 13 countries

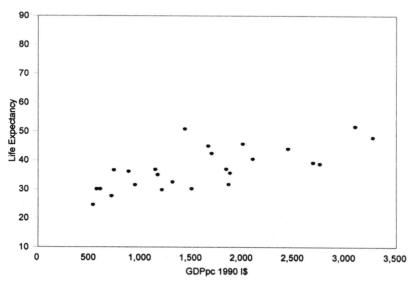

(b) 1870: 25 countries

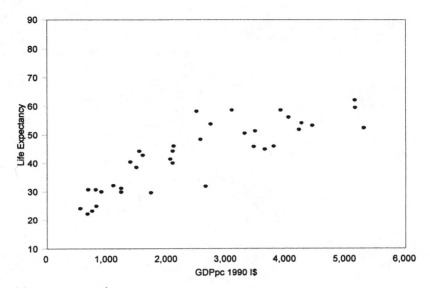

(c) 1913: 37 countries

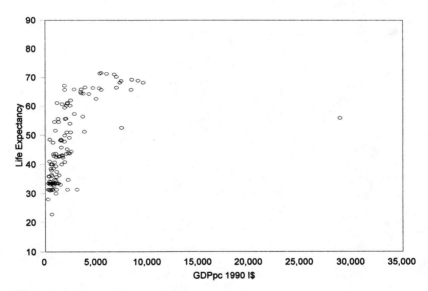

(d) 1950: 126 countries

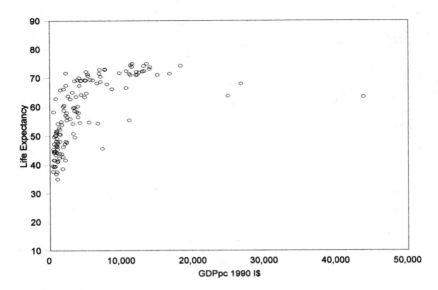

(e) 1973: 132 countries

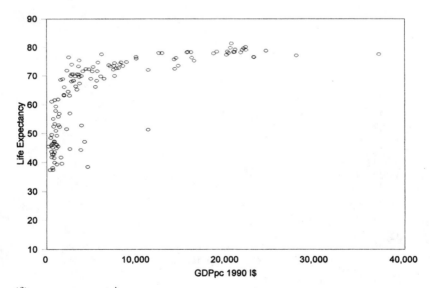

(f) 2001: 132 countries

SOURCES: Angus Maddison, *The World Economy: Historical Statistics* (Paris: Development Center of the Organization for Economic Cooperation and Development, 2003), pp. 58–69, 87–89, 100–101, 142–48, 180–87, 218–23; and James C. Riley, "Bibliography of Works Providing Estimates of Life Expectancy at Birth and of the Beginning Period of Health Transitions in Countries with a Population in 2000 of at least 400,000" at www.lifetable .de/RileyBib.htm, with comments on sources preferred for certain estimates.

If the assumption is made that cause runs more strongly from income to life expectancy than from life expectancy to income, then one implication of this analysis is that a higher income level was most effective in promoting higher life expectancy between 1870 and 1913. That was the beginning period of investments by the richer lands in water filtration and chlorination and in sewage treatment and disposal, which controlled many water-borne diseases, and of investments in education, mostly in primary schooling, which armed the general population with ways to inform themselves about disease risks. Considering the possibility of an association running from superior health to superior income, however, it may also be true that gains in survival in that period had a positive effect on labor productivity.[21]

The association between income per capita and life expectancy remained strong in 2001, intensified by the rising number of African countries with low income and low life expectancy. But it had less strength then than it had had at any earlier year back to 1820.

Table 4 shows results from the linear analysis of income change and life expectancy change *between* each pair of dates. Two comparisons—1870 to 1913 and 1950 to 1973—stand out, showing a positive association between the *pace* (percentage) of income growth and of life expectancy gains and between the *amount* of income growth and life expectancy gains, though in both cases only the latter association is statistically significant. In the 1820 to 1870 comparison, which includes only eleven cases, ten of them from Europe, income gains coincided with life expectancy losses often enough to produce a negative association. For 1913 to 1950 neither the pace nor the amount of income change was positively associated with life expectancy gains often enough to show up as statistically significant. The association present from 1950 to 1973 broke down in the succeeding comparison, between 1973 and 2001, a period when many countries lost life expectancy and also when life expectancy gains coincided with losses in income in some countries.

Of course income, by itself, does not produce higher survival odds or better health. Countries and families with higher incomes have the advantage that they can elect to spend more on health or seek out health-favoring investments, such as the water filtration and piping systems that European cities began to build in the late nineteenth century, which counterbalance some health-disfavoring factors, such as larger cities with denser populations, crowded housing, and a greater potential for contamination of water with human waste.

TABLE 3. Statistical Relationship between Income per Capita and Life Expectancy for 6 Periods (1820–2001) Shown in Figures 4a–f

	Number of Countries	Adjusted R-square	Without Outliers
1820	13	–.003	—
1870	25	.477***	—
1913	37	.720***	—
1950	126	.300***	.586***
1973	132	.335***	.557***
2001	132	.460***	—

SOURCES: Angus Maddison, *The World Economy: Historical Statistics* (Paris: Development Center of the Organization for Economic Cooperation and Development, 2003), pp. 33, 58–69, 87–89, 100–101, 111, 142–44, 147–48, 180–87, 218–24; James C. Riley, "Bibliography of Works Providing Estimates of Life Expectancy at Birth and of the Beginning Period of Health Transitions in Countries with a Population in 2000 of at least 400,000" at www.lifetable.de/RileyBib.htm.

*** significant at $p < .001$

Any discussion of the association between income and health thus requires two prior discussions. One of those deals with how much the people who make spending decisions, in the household or in the public sector, know about factors that favor health, how accurate their knowledge is, and how effectively they assess the efficiency of differing options in safeguarding or enhancing health. The other deals with the decisions actually made about spending, which are certain to be influenced by many other things than just the health-favoring qualities of one item that may be acquired compared to another. Thus, for example, visiting a doctor may be the most effective thing a householder can do for the recovery of a sick child, but the decision to visit may depend on many unrelated things: the doctor's proximity, whether there is still enough money left from the last paycheck to pay the doctor, the parents' judgment about how serious the sickness is, the implicit value the parents assign to that child, and many more.

This is not the place to attempt to construct a theory or a history of spending choices. Nevertheless the point being made can be buttressed by examining the association between UN estimates of per capita spending on health in 174 countries in 2001 and life expectancy in those countries, which appears in figure 5. This figure shows two distributions. Along

TABLE 4. Change in Income and in Life Expectancy, 1820–2001, Using Data from Table 3

	Number of Countries	Adjusted R-square, Percentage Income Change and Life Expectancy Change	Adjusted R-square, Amount of Income Change and Life Expectancy Change
1820–70	11	−.100	−.099
1870–1913	25	.090	.323**
1913–50	37	−.025	.009
1950–73	127	.001	.127***
1973–2001	133	.008	−.007

SOURCES: Angus Maddison, *The World Economy: Historical Statistics* (Paris: Development Center of the Organization for Economic Cooperation and Development, 2003), pp. 33, 58–69, 87–89, 100–101, 111, 142–44, 147–48, 180–87, 218–24; James C. Riley, "Bibliography of Works Providing Estimates of Life Expectancy at Birth and of the Beginning Period of Health Transitions in Countries with a Population in 2000 of at least 400,000" at www.lifetable.de/RileyBib.htm.

NOTE: Because the data are incomplete and the analyses consider differing time comparisons, the number of countries considered in this table differs slightly from the number in Table 3.

** significant at $p < .01$; *** significant at $p < .001$

the vertical axis many countries in 2001 spent less on health than U.S.$ (of 2001) 500 per capita, combining public and private spending, amid radically different life expectancy levels, ranging from less than 35 years to more than 75. And along the horizontal axis life expectancies clustered in the area about 70 years and above, even though per capita spending varied from less than $500 to nearly $5,000 (in the United States). Clearly in some countries, such as the United States, people and policymakers appear to have made massively ineffectual decisions about how to spend money on health services. And, at the other extreme, countries varied little in their spending per capita, but widely in the life expectancy level. Even though a statistical analysis suggests an association between health spending and life expectancy level, nearly all of the association will have to be explained by other factors.[22]

It is also evident, from the comparative study of national histories, that different countries have typically followed different paths in elevating life expectancies. Those paths were determined by the options available when one country's health transition began, by what the people in a country and its public sector could afford to do, and most especially by which of the many opportunities for action were seized. In a well-known exam-

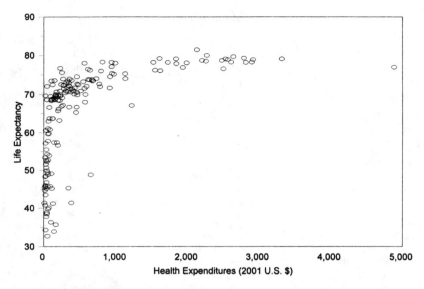

FIGURE 5. Life expectancy and per capita spending on health in 174 countries in 2001.
SOURCE: United Nations, Human Development Report 2004, at http://hdr
.undp.org/statistics/data/indic/indic_52_1_1.html, accessed July 8, 2005.

ple, Japan, which invested little in sanitary improvements, did not follow the same path as Britain, which invested heavily in sanitary improvements.[23] The same thing is true in nearly every comparison, and it is this variety in paths followed and opportunities seized that motivated the research behind this book.

All the countries considered in this study, the twelve given extended treatment and the others discussed briefly, share the characteristic of getting a bigger survival pay-off for what consumers and the public sector spent on health and health-related items than did the United States or other high-income countries. But it may be more important to look not so much at how they spent their money as at other things that were largely independent of income. In the case studies that begin with chapter 3 the issue of income will regularly be raised. But most of the discussion in those case studies deals with actions taken in lieu of spending, for the main point is that in these countries people were too poor simply to spend their way into better health.

Conclusion

Sustained economic growth began before sustained gains in survival. All the countries that initiated health transitions before 1900 began the process of elevating life expectancy when they were low-income lands, judged by the standards of the period 1950–present: that is, they were all poor by today's standards (although they were already richer than many of the low-income countries of the years 1950–present). The evidence reviewed in this chapter suggests that it has been difficult for countries to initiate and sustain gains in survival from GDPpc levels below I$ 1,000 in 1990 values, a threshold that seems to distinguish the health transition pioneers from other countries and regions. (In international dollars of 2005, the threshold would be roughly 1,500.) Above that threshold, however, income levels in the nineteenth century did not determine either the level of life expectancy or the period when gains in survival might begin.

Among countries with per capita incomes above I$ 1,000, income itself seems to have held little importance in 1820. The average income level began to matter in life expectancy gains between 1820 and 1870, and in 1913 the association between income and life expectancy levels peaked. Yet some countries attained higher incomes for that period, well above I$ 1,000, before they managed to begin health transitions.

To this point scholarly investigations of life expectancy gains in nineteenth-century Europe have focused on improvements in nutrition and public health. Sköld's work on the virtual eradication of smallpox in Sweden early in the nineteenth century suggests that additional factors may also be important. For Sweden's control of smallpox, social organization and political will mattered more than income, and it may be that this explanation offers a clue for understanding why the pioneer countries in general were able to elevate life expectancy.

In other respects, however, the experience of the pioneers offers less promise of providing answers to the question of how some low-income lands were able to begin their own health transitions and sustain those transitions to the point that they matched the rich countries in life expectancy. The threshold of I$ 1,000 in 1990 values may be important and will be considered in the case studies that follow. But the point at which income growth was initiated and the changing association between income and life expectancy levels will not matter, at least for the low-income countries that remained poor. More especially, the investments that Western countries made, such as in urban public health improvements, will not matter because none of the countries to be considered in this study could afford to follow that path.

Moreover, spending on health appears to be weakly related to life expectancy, at least around 2001. Some countries do an ineffectual job in their spending and some countries an excellent job of it, assessed by survival and therefore by the proportion of people at each age in their populations living through that year of life. The most interesting cases are those doing an exceptionally good job of it.

CHAPTER 2

Which Countries Should Be Studied?

Examining the Data

The roster of low- and middle-income countries with high life expectancy changes from time to time. Which cases should be studied? One place to begin in finding an answer to this question is the present. As of 2000 the countries of the world were distributed across a spectrum in GDPpc running from very low to very high levels. There are no obvious thresholds at which to distinguish low- from middle- from high-income countries. Figure 6 shows GDPpc in 2000 for the 130 countries for which Angus Maddison provides estimates, all in 1990 international dollars, across the range from I$ 218 for the Congo Democratic Republic to I$ 28,129 for the United States. Using the discontinuities that appear in this diagram, table 5 shows one plausible set of income groupings. The lowest group can be further divided, and one possibility is to distinguish countries with GDPpc levels under I$ 1,000 from those with levels between I$ 1,000 and 5,000. This distribution provides a useful way to distinguish among countries according to how far the GDPpc level might be expected to contribute to life expectancy gains as of 2000, but it gives no assistance in extending this expectation back in time.

Figure 7 distributes countries by GDPpc in PPP or international dollars for 2000 and life expectancy for the same year, using United Nations statistics and shows both global and regional distributions. Comparing this figure with figure 4f (in chapter 1), which uses the life expectancy estimates I assembled plus Maddison's GDPpc estimates in 1990 I$, will show a close resemblance between the two and distributions with the same shape.

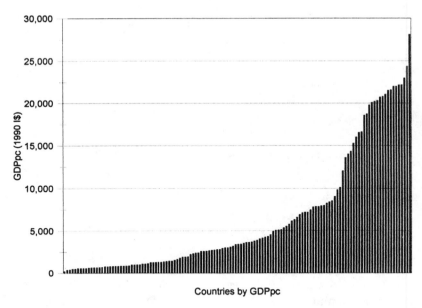

Countries by GDPpc

FIGURE 6. Gross domestic product per capita (GDPpc) in 1990 international dollars (I$) in 2000 for 130 countries.
SOURCE: Angus Maddison, *The World Economy: Historical Statistics* (Paris: Development Center of the Organization for Economic Cooperation and Development, 2003), pp. 64–65, 69, 89, 101, 144, 147–48, 184–87, and 218–23.

TABLE 5. Grouping of the 130 Countries in Figure 6 by Gross Domestic Product per Capita (GDPpc) as of 2000

Income Level	GDPpc (1990 international dollars)	Number of Countries
High	18,596 and above	18
Middle	9,841–16,642	10
Low: group a	5,065–9,047	23
Low: group b	5,000 and below	79
b1	1,000–5,000	52
b2	below 1,000	27

SOURCE: Angus Maddison, *The World Economy: Historical Statistics* (Paris: Development Center of the Organization for Economic Cooperation and Development, 2003), pp. 64–65, 69, 87, 89, 105, 111, 142, 144, 146–49, 218–24.

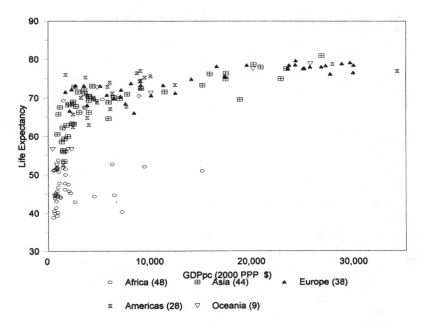

FIGURE 7. Gross domestic product per capita GDPpc in 2000 PPP dollars and life expectancy in 2000 for 167 countries.
SOURCES: United Nations Development Programme, *Human Development Report 2002* (New York: Oxford University Press, 2002), pp. 149–52; also A. D. Lopez et al., *World Mortality in 2000: Life Tables for 191 Countries* (Geneva: World Health Organization, 2002); and United States, Central Intelligence Agency, World Factbook, at www.odci.gov/cia/publications/factbook/index.html, accessed various dates in 2003.

Some countries have lower levels of life expectancy than seem to be warranted by their income levels; they are sometimes called under-achievers.[1] Other countries have higher levels of life expectancy than seem to be warranted, and, once again, they are the most interesting cases for this study. These countries appear in the upper left corner, in the elbow, of the distribution in figures 7 and 4f. They are listed in table 6, using an expansive definition, including all countries for which, first, Maddison estimates GDPpc in 2000 below I$ 7,250 and, second, from my database, life expectancy at birth is estimated at or above 65 years.[2] As of 2000, as we have seen, all the high-income countries had high survival rates, even though the distribution of income per capita and life expectancy among them does not suggest that the highest income can be associated with the

TABLE 6. Countries with High Life Expectancies but Low Incomes in 2000

	Gross Domestic Product per capita[a]	Life Expectancy[b]
Albania	2,807	74.0
Algeria	2,792	71.0
Bahrain	5,065	73.1
Brazil	5,556	68.1
Bulgaria	5,365	71.6
Cape Verde	1,777	68.8
China	3,425	70.3
Colombia	5,096	71.6
Costa Rica	6,174	77.5
Cuba	2,414	76.5
Dominican Republic	3,663	67.3
Ecuador	3,101	69.6
Egypt	2,920	67.5
El Salvador	2,716	70.2
Guatemala	3,396	65.2
Honduras	1,957	66.0
Hungary	7,138	71.3
Indonesia	3,203	66.0
Iran	4,911	69.1
Jamaica	3,548	75.3
Jordan	4,055	71.5
Lebanon	3,430	70.4
Libya	2,322	71.0
Mexico	7,218	73.0

highest life expectancy. The surest path to high life expectancy has been becoming a high-income country. But the low- and middle-income countries do not uniformly have lower survival rates.

It is not just the situation of 2000 that should be allowed to determine whether a country warrants study for combining low income with high life expectancy, however. Figure 8 shows the distribution of GDPpc and life expectancy in the period of initiation of health transitions for the 89 countries for which both pieces of information are available. (This figure excludes one outlier, Kuwait, which at the beginning of its health transition, when oil exports produced an explosive surge in income, had a GDPpc of nearly I$ 29,000 and a life expectancy of 26.) Up to the 1890s

TABLE 6. (*continued*)

	Gross Domestic Product per capita[a]	Life Expectancy[b]
Morocco	2,658	67.5
Nicaragua	1,558	68.9
Oman	6,926	73.6
Panama	5,782	74.6
Paraguay	3,014	70.4
Peru	3,686	69.3
Philippines	2,385	69.3
Poland	7,215	73.3
Romania	3,002	69.9
Russia	5,157	65.3
Sri Lanka	3,645	73.1
Thailand	6,336	68.8
Tunisia	4,538	72.1
Turkey	6,597	69.7
Ukraine	2,736	68.3
Yugoslavia	4,258	72.5

SOURCES: Angus Maddison, *The World Economy: Historical Statistics* (Paris: Development Center of the Organization for Economic Cooperation and Development, 2003), pp. 33, 58–69, 87–89, 100–101, 111, 142–44, 147–48, 180–87, 218–24; James C. Riley, "Bibliography of Works Providing Estimates of Life Expectancy at Birth and of the Beginning Period of Health Transitions in Countries with a Population in 2000 of at least 400,000" at www.lifetable.de/RileyBib.htm.

[a]Low income is defined as less than 1990 international dollars 7,250.

[b]High life expectancy is defined as over 65 years.

only Canada, as has been remarked, began a health transition with a GDPpc level below I$ 1,000. In the twentieth century many more countries managed to do that. Although the I$ 1,000 threshold held up until the 1940s, most of the countries that began health transitions in the 1940s and 1950s had significantly lower levels of GDPpc. For the large group of countries that began transitions in the 1930s, 1940s, 1950s, or later (in the Appendix, from Burundi to the end), life expectancy in the beginning period averaged 32.7 years, not much different from the average of 33.1 years in the beginning period of all health transitions. But the GDPpc level dropped to an average of I$ 814. Some countries even managed to begin health transitions at times when their GDPpc, according to Maddison's estimates, was below I$ 400.

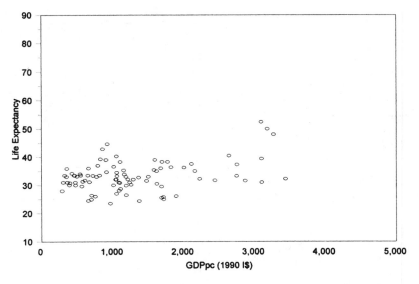

FIGURE 8. Distribution of gross domestic product per capita (GDPpc) in 1990 international dollars (I$) and life expectancy at the initiation of health transitions.
SOURCES: Angus Maddison, *The World Economy: Historical Statistics* (Paris: Development Center of the Organization for Economic Cooperation and Development, 2003), pp. 58–69, 87–89, 100–101, 142–48, 180–87, 218–23; and James C. Riley, "Bibliography of Works Providing Estimates of Life Expectancy at Birth and of the Beginning Period of Health Transitions in Countries with a Population in 2000 of at least 400,000" at www.lifetable.de/RileyBib.htm.

Antibiotics and Vaccinations

Something intervened, in the 1940s or early 1950s, to allow persistent gains in life expectancy to begin at a lower income level. The most widely held assumption about what was new in this period points to new medicines, especially antibiotics, and vaccines. Penicillin and other antibiotics began to reach the poorer countries in Africa, Asia, and Latin America in the late 1940s and early 1950s. For example, they arrived in Venezuela, a country with close contacts to the United States, in 1950.[3] Vaccines spread more slowly, and that was true not just of the established vaccines for smallpox and typhoid fever but also the new vaccines introduced in the 1950s and 1960s. In most countries that began health transitions between the 1890s and the 1920s or 1930s, however, mortality from diseases treatable with antibiotics, such as tuberculosis and typhoid fever, was already much reduced by the time the antibiotics became available. That was true also for the countries that began health transitions before the 1890s. Thus the effects posited for antibiotics apply chiefly to countries where bacterial infections remained leading causes of death, which would include all the countries shown in the Appendix that initiated health transitions in the 1940s or later. Antibiotics, and to a much lesser degree sulfa drugs especially effective in treating wounds and sores, are said to have allowed those countries to make rapid progress in controlling infectious diseases.

While it is plausible to suppose that antibiotics, sulfa drugs, and vaccines made it possible to begin health transitions without first achieving the level of economic development associated with per capita incomes above I$ 1,000, that idea has received remarkably little scrutiny. Few studies have been done on the actual dissemination of antibiotics and vaccines in the period 1945–60 in Africa, Asia, and Latin America. Many of the countries that began health transitions in the 1940s or 1950s had quite poorly developed healthcare and public health systems, with few hospitals, few physicians and nurses trained in Western medicine, and few health centers, clinics, or dispensaries. If antibiotics and vaccines were in fact instrumental, one must imagine that they were distributed outside, or mostly outside, such systems. In addition, ordinary people must have learned quickly about these remedies, how to obtain them, and when and how to use them, and they must also have been able to afford the new medications and vaccines. Put that way, the proposition looks more doubtful. Did antibiotics actually reach large proportions of the populations of Africa, Asia, and Latin America by 1950, or even by 1960?

Whatever the case, there were significant survival gains across at least three decades, from the 1950s through the 1970s. Nearly all of the low-income countries that began health transitions between the 1890s and the 1920s or 1930s, before the availability of antibiotics or sulfa drugs, continued to add to those earlier gains in the period 1970–2000 as well. But many of the countries that began transitions in the 1940s or later saw their gains falter in the 1980s in the face of HIV/AIDS, tuberculosis (both drug-resistant and non-resistant strains), resurgent malaria, unresolved problems with fecal disease, and other communicable diseases. The steps taken toward improved survival among countries that initiated health transitions between the 1890s and the 1920s or 1930s seem to have laid a better foundation for long-run gains than did the antibiotics and vaccines deployed in the late 1940s and thereafter, or whatever other factors might be posited as having mattered.

For vaccinations there is also reason to be skeptical whether their effects were felt so early in low-income countries. Smallpox vaccination was introduced in England in 1796, as has already been noted. Although it was soon used in many different parts of the world, decades passed before usage was general in any large region in Africa, Asia, or Latin America. For example, in Sri Lanka vaccination was first used in 1802 but was not widely deployed until the 1890s. News of Jenner's vaccine reached Japan in 1803, and vaccine itself arrived in 1823, although that initial sample had lost its viability. But vaccination was not widely used until the 1870s. Even then, much slower progress was made in controlling smallpox in Japan than had been made in Sweden in the earliest decades of the nineteenth century: the last major epidemic in Japan occurred in 1897.[4] In sum, delays in the dissemination of smallpox vaccine were typical rather than unusual.

The same delay applied to other vaccines. A typhoid fever vaccine with an effectiveness of "about 75 per cent" was introduced in 1896.[5] But in Jamaica and Sri Lanka, to give two examples, it was the 1930s before the vaccine was used, and then only on a limited scale.[6] Mass vaccination for typhoid fever remained uncommon into the 1940s, when instead the antibiotic chloramphenical began to be used to treat this disease, at least in the West.

Thus the date when a vaccine was introduced in the West has little usefulness in determining when that vaccine was first used, or first widely used, in the developing world, where, in any case, the medical infrastructure was rarely developed enough to support mass immunizations. Vaccines with general or limited usefulness against smallpox, typhoid fever, yellow fever, certain forms of tuberculosis, tetanus, plague, and whooping cough were all introduced in the West before World War II, but only smallpox vaccination seems to have been used widely in some parts of the developing world before the 1940s. After the war vaccines for polio (introduced in 1954), measles (1963), mumps (1967), and rubella (1969) might have had a substantial and immediate effect, but it was the 1970s or even the 1980s before many of them were used widely. In the absence of a detailed reconstruction of the timing and scale of vaccine use, it is difficult to determine when they actually had a general effect. Except for smallpox, the answer is likely to be the 1970s and 1980s as part of the World Health Organization's Expanded Program on Immunization.[7]

In sum, although antibiotics and vaccinations may have helped initiate mortality declines in many countries in the 1940s and 1950s, it seems likelier that their effect was felt somewhat later and more weakly.

Choosing the Case Studies

So far two groups of countries have been excluded, or nearly so, in this search for ways to identify countries with good health but low income suitable for this study. First, even though the countries that pioneered health transitions between the 1770s and the 1880s were all low-income at the beginning point, most of them have been excluded from consideration because they became high-income countries so early. The second group so far excluded is made up of countries that began health transitions in the 1940s or thereafter, since too few of these countries managed to combine low income with substantial life expectancy gains. In fact, only five of the forty-eight countries in this category (see Appendix, Burundi to Oman) managed to elevate life expectancy to levels at or above 67 years. Three of those—Bahrain, Oman, and Saudi Arabia—were oil-rich countries and therefore exceptional cases. (The other two were the Solomon Islands, which attained a life expectancy of 68.6 years in 2000, and Mongolia, with 67 years in 2000.) Nor were these cases where high life expectancy was attained and then lost in the face of HIV/AIDS or any other cause. Thus this group of countries supplies only a few potential cases of low income but high life expectancy, the most interesting of which are the oil-rich lands. Chapter 8 will look at a larger group of oil-rich lands and explore the policies and strategies followed by countries in the peculiar circumstances of not having to consider cost nearly as carefully as other lands did.

As a result of these factors, the attention of this study focuses on the group of countries that initiated health transitions between the 1890s and the 1930s, and in particular on the ones among them that more or less matched the rich lands in life expectancy by the 1950s or 1960s. This approach means that some countries that went on to become rich lands (Japan) or high middle-income countries (South Korea) will be included as case studies. So will some that faltered in life expectancy improvement and also did not sustain economic growth at a rapid enough pace to become rich lands. Most of the countries formerly within the Soviet Union and many countries formerly part of the Soviet bloc fit this description. So do Suriname, Guyana, and North Korea. Nonetheless, some of these cases are worth examination, with most of the attention falling on the period of persistent gains in survival and on explanations for those gains. Chapter 7 considers in particular the Soviet Union / Russia and China, with some discussion of Albania and Ukraine.

Most of the chapters and case studies that follow, however, deal with lands that fit among the 2000 group of good-health-at-low-income countries. Not every country in this group will be considered in the same detail. Some that might have provided case studies, such as Puerto Rico and Kerala state in India, will be mentioned at points where parallels can be drawn rather than being treated in depth. Others, including Barbados, Fiji, Greece, Malaysia, Mauritius, Taiwan, and Vietnam, will not appear, chiefly because their histories are not yet well enough known to be summarized. Detailed case studies, then, will examine life expectancy progress in twelve countries: Japan and Korea; Sri Lanka; Panama and Costa Rica; Cuba and Jamaica; the Soviet Union and China; Oman; and Venezuela and Mexico.

Pioneers and the Group of Twelve

The case studies that follow relate the main features of the health transition in each of the group of twelve lands to be examined in some detail. The first point, to be discussed here, is to compare the twelve to the countries that pioneered health transitions on the basic issues of when, at what level of life expectancy, and at what level of GDPpc the transitions began. Tables 7 (the pioneer countries) and 8 (the group of twelve) show that the twelve began their health transitions about a century later than the pioneer countries and at roughly the same level of income per person, but at a significantly lower average level of survival. Yet they made more rapid progress, as has already been remarked. (These tables will be useful for the case studies that follow in chapters 3 through 9 because they allow comparisons among the group of twelve on these fundamental issues. Thus it may help the reader to attach a piece of sticky paper to the page with these two tables, the easier to refer back to them later.)

Still, comparison on these basic points is inadequate. Sweden's experience with smallpox vaccination shows that what matters in a country's capacity to initiate and sustain improvements in survival lies more in its capacity for social organization and growth than in its level of income. And France's rapid convergence toward the other pioneer countries in life expectancy, beginning at a significantly lower level, shows further that the beginning survival level is less important than a country's capacity to mobilize resources for improvement.

Thus the main point of the case studies that follow is to identify what resources countries in the group of twelve substituted for modernization and development in the style followed by the countries that pioneered

TABLE 7. Basic Information about Countries That Pioneered Health Transitions

	Initiation of Health Transition	Life Expectancy at Initiation	Gross Domestic Product per Capita at Initiation (1990 international dollars)
Denmark	1770s	about 33	1,186[a]
France	1790s	28.1	1,088[a]
Sweden	1790s	35.3	1,152[a]
England and Wales	1800s	36.3 (England only)	2,006 (England and Wales plus Scotland)
Norway	1810s	38.3	1,104
Canada	1820s or 1830s	39.0	904
Belgium	1840s	38.3	1,694
average	about 1810	35.5	1,305

SOURCE: James C. Riley, "The Timing and Pace of Health Transitions around the World," *Population and Development Review* 31 (2005): 758–64.

[a]Interpolating between dates for which estimates are given.

TABLE 8. Basic Information about the Group of Twelve

	Initiation of Health Transition	Life Expectancy at Initiation	Gross Domestic Product per Capita at Initiation (1990 international dollars)
Mexico	1860s to 1890	24–29	1,189
Japan	1870s to 1890s	36.6 (1870)	1,012
Russia	1890s or 1900s	31 (1897)	1,237
Costa Rica	1890s to 1920s	30.5 (1890s) to 33.3–34.1 (1920s)	1,624 (1920)
Cuba	1900s	33.1–38.4	n.a.
Korea	1910s	23.5	966
Panama	1910s	n.a.	1,258 (1926)[a]
China	1920s	24.2–35	562 (1929)
Jamaica	1920s	37.0	789[b]
Sri Lanka	1920s	29.9 (1911)	1,187
Venezuela	1920s or 1930s	32.2 (1926)	3,444
Oman	1940s to 1970s	40.3	1,053
average	about 1915	32.1	1,400

SOURCES: Angus Maddison, *The World Economy: Historical Statistics* (Paris: Development Center of the Organization for Economic Cooperation and Development, 2003), pp. 100, 114, 142–46, 160–61, 186; James C. Riley, "The Timing and Pace of Health Transitions around the World," *Population and Development Review* 31 (2005): 758–64.

[a]Interpolating from Maddison's estimate for countries in the region to his estimate for Panama alone.

[b]Interpolating between dates for which estimates are given.

health transitions. Each narrative has been organized around the proposition of showing the level and pace of economic development in order to rule out gains in income until they actually occurred. Stripping out income growth, what remains is the story about these twelve.

Conclusion

This chapter has explained the selection process and identified the countries selected for closer study. The chapters that follow provide succinct histories of life expectancy and attempt to explain survival gains in each of this wide-ranging group of good-health-at-low-income countries. They deal with countries that initiated health transitions between the 1890s and the 1920s or 1930s, before the availability of antibiotics and most vaccines, plus a group of countries made suddenly wealthy by oil that initiated health transitions as late as the 1950s, 1960s, or 1970s. Each case study relies on the knowledge that specialists have acquired about the factors that matter the most. Each will show many distinctive, or even unique factors, and some common elements. The main goal in each case is to understand how so many countries managed to make substantial and significant progress in controlling survival in the period between 1890 and 1960.

These case studies are organized around both chronological and topical lines. They begin in Asia with two of the earlier health transitions, in Japan and Korea, and then move forward in time and from Asia to the Americas and the Caribbean, Europe, and then to the Middle East and North Africa, ending up with the Middle East and Oman, which initiated improvements in survival last among all the countries considered. The last chapter returns to the Americans to consider Mexico and a particular issue: How did one country with a marked disparity in the distribution of income and wealth manage nevertheless to begin and sustain a health transition?

CHAPTER 3

A Colonizer and the Country Colonized

Japan and Korea

Japan and South Korea both broke out of the ranks of low-income countries in the post–World War II era. Although Japan had made considerable progress in economic development in the period 1870–1940, exceptionally rapid economic growth began only at the end of the 1940s. In South Korea similarly rapid growth started in the 1960s (figure 9).[1]

Both countries had initiated health transitions much earlier, Japan between the 1870s and 1890s, probably in the 1890s, and Korea in the 1910s, while under Japanese occupation that began in 1906 (figure 10).[2] Figure 11 shows period-to-period change in life expectancy, including Japan's losses during World War II and its rapid recovery afterward. Both countries made unusually rapid gains in survival from the 1910s. For Korea those rapid gains persisted up to World War II, which brought hard times but not active combat. Survival then plunged during the Korean War, but gains resumed after that conflict and ended at about the same time that rapid economic gains began. Japan curtailed its survival gains in the late 1920s, as it shifted resources to a military build-up, but from about 1947 into the 1970s enjoyed irregular but mostly substantial year-to-year progress, which up to 1975 averaged nearly two-thirds of a year added to life expectancy at birth for each year of calendar time. Around 1978 Japan took the global lead in life expectancy from Sweden.[3]

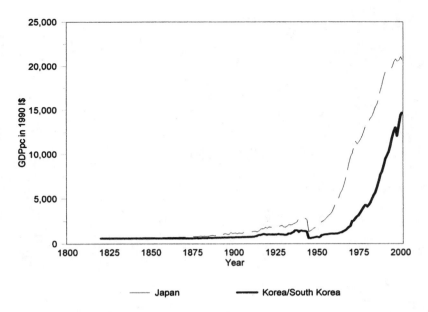

FIGURE 9. Gross domestic product per capita (GDPpc) in 1990 international dollars (I$) in Japan and Korea / South Korea, 1820–2001.
SOURCE: Angus Maddison, *The World Economy: Historical Statistics* (Paris: Development Center of the Organization for Economic Cooperation and Development, 2003), pp. 180, 182, and 184.

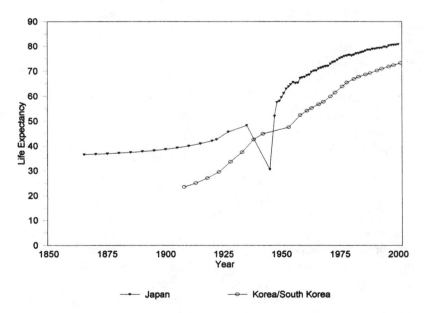

FIGURE 10. Life expectancy in Japan and Korea / South Korea, 1865–2000.
SOURCE: James C. Riley, "Bibliography of Works Providing Estimates of Life Expectancy at Birth and of the Beginning Period of Health Transitions in Countries with a Population in 2000 of at least 400,000" at www.lifetable .de/RileyBib.htm.

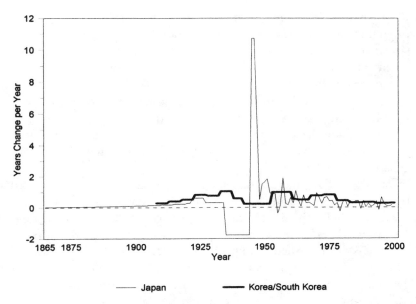

FIGURE 11. Pace of change in life expectancy in Japan and Korea / South Korea, 1865–2000.
SOURCE: James C. Riley, "Bibliography of Works Providing Estimates of Life Expectancy at Birth and of the Beginning Period of Health Transitions in Countries with a Population in 2000 of at least 400,000" at www.lifetable .de/RileyBib.htm.

Japan

At some point before the 1720s Japan seems to have moved from the high-mortality situation found in most Neolithic societies to comparatively high survival rates and a life expectancy in the 30s, roughly equivalent to England's in the same period. Susan Hanley and Alan Macfarlane explain Japan's high survival by pointing to low-cost but healthy housing and hygienic lifestyles, which included regular bathing and drinking tea prepared with boiled water.[4] However, the nutritional status of the Japanese, whether assessed by stature or by elements of diet, remained marginal, and nutritional diseases such as beriberi continued to cause some deaths into the 1920s.

Thus Japanese in the Tokugawa period (1615–1868) enjoyed high survival, at least in its latter half, compared to other global regions of that era, although this did not actually initiate, or lay foundations for, a health transition. Social policy may also have contributed to the advantage under the Tokugawa government, which implemented a rudimentary welfare program that included poorhouses for disabled people and a mutual aid system. Considering the effect of this system, Toshiyuki Mizoguchi and Noriyuki Takayama conclude "that the standard of living of the people was low with relatively equal income distribution."[5]

In most versions the history of Japan's health transition begins with the Meiji Restoration of 1868, which initiated substantial changes in the organization of the government; the adaptation of Western institutions to Japanese uses; the use of Western technologies, including smallpox vaccination from 1876–78; schooling and literacy; and economic development. The new regime also maintained the welfare practices introduced by its predecessor, but these continued to provide relief to only a small fraction of the population. In the early years of the Meiji era (1868–1912) Japan made laws before it really had the capacity to enforce them. When practice is distinguished from plan, the adoption of Western ideas and practices certainly made more headway in medicine and economic development than in education.[6] New physicians were increasingly trained in Western rather than Chinese medicine, but Japan also elected to train many doctors for a few years rather than to follow the German model of protracted and increasingly specialized training. Medical services were deployed to benefit children, such as via smallpox vaccinations, rather than to care for the aged. Throughout this phase of Japan's mortality decline, up to the 1940s, most deaths occurred without medical attendance.[7]

Japan controlled cholera by quarantines, introduced in the 1870s. But smallpox and cholera are the only two diseases against which progress was clearly being made before 1900. By 1900 Japan's profile of causes of death resembled that in West European countries, with important exceptions. As in Western Europe, the leading causes of death were respiratory and chronic diseases. But in Japan mortality from typhoid fever and other diarrheal diseases remained heavy, and tuberculosis persisted as a leading cause of death.[8] In 1937 the country claimed, among some 13.8 million households, not quite 87,000 with modernized means of waste disposal, mostly in Tokyo. In the same year only 26 percent of houses were connected to public waterworks, the proportion being as high as 70 percent in Tokyo but only 5 percent in rural districts.[9] Typhoid fever, which caused as many as 16.2 deaths per 100,000 people in 1926 and 10 in 1940, was not brought under control until 1947.[10] Tuberculosis mortality increased with industrialization and urbanization, up to the 1920s, and remained high until after World War II, a distinct break with the pattern in Western Europe, the United States, and Canada, where mortality from tuberculosis began to decline in the nineteenth century.

In education more was done initially to conceptualize than to implement reforms. The initial Meiji plan was to translate Western texts, including some on science and hygiene, into Japanese for use in the schools. That plan was shelved by 1880, and the curriculum actually implemented featured moral exhortation and nationalism more than Western technical material.[11] Compulsory schooling for four years was ordered in 1886. (Most authorities believe that four years of schooling is enough to provide basic literacy and to train children in the school culture with its discipline, group activities, and points of indoctrination.) Japan's compulsory schooling law was effectively enforced by 1911, assisted by a 1900 decision to drop tuition, which persuaded many farmers to send their children to school.[12] Meiji reforms called upon the schools to teach hygiene lessons taken from Western texts, and the government organized campaigns to reform popular habits, some with health themes.[13] But more research will be required to determine how effective these programs may have been. Literacy certainly improved, rising for males from perhaps 35 percent in the 1860s to 75 percent in the 1910s, and for females from 8 to 68 percent across the same period.[14]

Women continued to occupy a subordinate place in public life, but female school enrollments rose and drop-out rates fell across the period 1881–1940.[15] Meiji era schools educated women for roles as good wives and mothers, which in fact gave them more authority within the household than they had had in the preceding Tokugawa period.[16]

Between about 1900 and 1930 a new middle class emerged, made up mostly of civil servants, educators, managers, office workers, and professionals—people who depended on their education and technical skills. This group adopted some Western ideas about the home and conjugal family, sought to improve home life and domestic happiness, and practiced frugality.[17]

In the Meiji era Japanese economic growth likewise made headway, building on Tokugawa era advances in technology, trade, and commercial agriculture. But Japan remained far poorer than its European counterparts. Its 1900 GDPpc (in constant values) surpassed its 1870 level by 60 percent, but was only 26 percent as large as that of the United Kingdom.[18] Early Japanese industrialization ignored consequences for the urban environment, sanitation, disease, and pollution.[19] The distribution of income became more skew across the period 1890 to 1920, which suggests that working people had less opportunity to invest in health than rising levels of average per capita income might indicate.[20]

On the eve of World War II, when life expectancy for males equaled 46.9 years and for females 49.6 years, Japan possessed an incomplete health infrastructure. Its strongest points were the widespread use of small-pox vaccination; a large number of medical personnel; improving health care for infants and children and wide distribution of information about infant care; effective quarantines and the surveillance and containment of many infectious diseases; food and milk inspection; plus the helpful habits and attitudes of the populace. Its weakest points lay in an incomplete system for delivering pure water and disposing of waste; urban crowding, poor nutrition, and persistently high rates of tuberculosis mortality; and the government's militaristic orientation, which produced life-wasting rather than life-saving policies.[21]

After World War II Japan added years of survival at an extraordinarily rapid pace.[22] In the early postwar years survivorship improved most among the young. Yet Japan gained its life expectancy lead over other industrial countries not just by pushing the mortality of the young down but also by achieving very low mortality for the old. From the latter 1980s lower mortality among people aged 65 and over contributed the largest share of all gains. Thus the postwar period itself can be divided into two parts. In the first, which lasted into the 1960s and benefited chiefly infants, children, and young adults, most of the gain came from lower death rates from tuberculosis, gastroenteritis and other fecal diseases, bronchitis, and pneumonia. Tuberculosis accounted for more than 200 deaths per 100,000 before the war. After the war mortality from this disease declined to fewer than 45 deaths per 100,000 in 1955 and only 8.5 in 1976 amid a national program of screening, vaccination with bacille Calmette-Guérin (BCG), and the widespread use of antibiotics. Quite quickly, by 1955, Japan reached a position in which the three leading causes of death were organ diseases associated with older ages: cerebrovascular disease (stroke), neoplasms (cancer), and heart disease. After 1965 gains were concentrated among adults and in lower death rates from cerebrovascular disease.[23]

The postwar retreat of mortality in Japan was assisted by a decisive shift of public resources away from military spending (which was capped by the new constitution at a maximum of 1 percent of national product) and toward health, welfare, and education. Japan expanded the number and responsibilities of its public health centers, assigning to them the task of monitoring the public's health, promoting sanitation reforms, providing health education, and also offering medical services. As in the prewar period, Japan for some time focused on providing more numerous rather than more highly trained doctors: the ratio of physicians engaged in medical practice per 100,000 people rose from 79.1 in 1948 to 103.8 in 1965 and 169.9 in 1992. Public authorities also took advantage of the population's cooperative attitude, introducing a series of national programs to screen for and treat leading causes of death, beginning with tuberculosis and continuing in the 1960s with cancer and stroke. Those campaigns paid off with high levels of public utilization and, in the case of tuberculosis and stroke but not cancer, noteworthy gains in disease control. Piped water and sewerage disposal systems were extended, but remained incomplete; even in 1990 only 43.7 percent of the population lived in districts connected to the sewerage system.[24] School feeding programs improved the nutrition of children, but for several years after 1947 calorie intake remained below the standard requirement.

To explain low infant mortality in the period 1950–85, Eikichi Matsuyama stresses the good health habits that Japanese mothers learned from their wide use of handbooks on maternal and child health. Central and local government agencies, private organizations, and the efforts of many mothers steadily produced healthier pregnancies, safer births, and better living conditions for early life. Also, few women delivered outside of marriage or at very young ages.[25]

Postwar economic growth assisted these improvements. So did more effective political institutions that were dedicated to improving survival, and the collaboration of the general population in public health programs. Economic growth also put additional resources into the hands of consumers, who made some purchases that reduced health risks. Between the late 1950s and 1965 Japanese consumers outfitted their homes with refrigerators, which had the beneficial effect of reducing demand for foods preserved with salt while increasing the consumption of fresh foods.[26] Postwar Japan benefited also from certain structural advantages, in addition to the high levels of literacy achieved before World War II and the readiness of its people to cooperate with government initiatives. Unemployment remained low. Income advanced: Japan jumped from a per capita GDP only 0.28 that of the United Kingdom in 1950 to 1.06 the level of the United Kingdom in 2000.[27] Japan's population moved into cities, where the concentration of public health and medical resources made death rates lower.[28] And in the postwar period inequality in income distribution diminished from the higher level maintained across the period 1920–40, with a Gini coefficient of 0.45 to 0.47, toward the range 0.33 to 0.37 maintained across the period 1962–82.[29]

The Gini coefficient provides a convenient gauge of inequality in the distribution of income, with values closer to zero indicating closer proximity to absolute equality, in which every individual or household has the same income or the same level of consumption, and higher values, approaching 1, indicating progressively less equality.[30] Anthony Atkinson and fellow authors surveyed the high-income countries in the Organization for Economic Cooperation and Development in the mid-1980s, finding a spread from Finland with the least inequality (a Gini coefficient of 0.21), to the United States with the most (a coefficient of 0.34).[31] In assessments across the twentieth and early twenty-first centuries, most countries fall within a wider range, from close to 0.20, as found in northwestern Europe, to about 0.60, as found in many Latin American countries.

Income distribution may influence survival in at least two ways. In the 1970s, G. B. Rodgers used income distribution estimates for fifty-six countries, including low- and high-income countries, to examine the relationship among income per capita, income distribution, and life expectancy. He found that "the difference in average life expectancy between a relatively egalitarian and a relatively inegalitarian country is likely to be as much as five to ten years."[32] And he associated inequality in the distribution of income with inequality in access to health services, education, and other factors associated with survival. Richard Wilkinson approached the issue in a different way in the 1990s. Restricting his study to already developed countries and to the attempt to explain why they differ in life expectancy, infant mortality, and other indices of health, he arrived at a more specific argument: "Health is related to differences in living standards within developed societies but not to the differences between them. . . . What matters within countries is relative rather than absolute income levels." In societies with less pronounced differentials, Wilkinson argues, there is greater social cohesion, death rates associated with crime and violence are lower, and risks associated with psychosocial dissonance and stress are milder.[33]

Wilkinson represented Japan as one of five examples of societies with less inequality in income distribution, greater social cohesion, and higher survival, associating Japan's move to a more even distribution of income with its attainment of the position of having the highest life expectancy of any large country.[34] Whether Japan has "the narrowest income differentials of any country," as Wilkinson maintains, depends on whether one measures differentiation before or after taxes and transfers.[35] If the assessment is before, then he may be correct; if afterwards, then decisively not: on the afterwards measure the Nordic lands all have significantly lower Gini coefficients.[36]

Japan's income distribution did become less uneven during World War II and in the immediate postwar years, and it may be that this adjustment should be associated with the rapid postwar recovery of survival. But from 1951 to 2002 the distribution remained roughly stable while survival improved continually in circumstances in which mortality from communicable (e.g., tuberculosis and typhoid fever) and noncommunicable diseases (coronary and cerebrovascular disease) diminished. If an association is to be drawn there, the argument must be not that inequality declined, as Wilkinson maintains, but that a stable if not especially egalitarian level of income distribution should be associated with improved life expectancy. And indeed, in the postwar period life expectancy rose in the poorest areas as well as in wealthier regions, and for much of that period the highest life expectancy occurred in Okinawa, the poorest prefecture.

Japan thus began to build high life expectancy following a substantially different path than the countries of Western Europe. In the early decades of its health transition Japan controlled cholera not through sanitation improvements but by quarantine, and only slowly, over many decades, did it move to piping water into and removing human waste from households. Tuberculosis mortality declined in many Western countries in the latter nineteenth century, but continued to rise during Japan's industrialization and militarization, into World War II. Japanese income increased after 1870, but more slowly than in Western countries. Even in 1950 the Japanese remained poorly nourished by the standards of stature and of nutritional disease, long after that had ceased to be the case for people in most Western countries.

Korea and South Korea

Although Doo-Sub Kim and Cheong-Seok Kim suggest that mortality in Korea began to decline around 1900, most authorities point to the early years of Japanese colonization, either the 1910s or 1920s, as the beginning point.[37] Japan extended its authority in Korea across the period 1876–1910 as part of an expansionist foreign policy that challenged Russian economic influence in this largely agrarian country that also had important iron and coal reserves. Many aspects of Korean experience as a Japanese colony mimicked developments in Japan. Although the Japanese fostered industrialization and agricultural output rose, there was not much improvement in living conditions, and for farmers, the most common occupation, conditions actually deteriorated. The "Japanese system" for public health, implemented in the years after 1906, featured quarantines, sanitary regulations, smallpox vaccination, and more widely available medical care, all of which helped reduce mortality by controlling infectious diseases. Japan built new hospitals in Korea, opened medical schools, and trained more physicians. The process of disease suppression was slow and uncertain, however. Japanese colonial authorities managed to control smallpox and cholera, epidemics of both diseases in 1920 notwithstanding. But there was a continuing heavy mortality from fecal disease and other diseases of the digestive system.[38] In addition, Sherwood Hall, a Canadian medical missionary who arrived in 1926, observed that "tuberculosis was sweeping unchecked through the country." Hall's efforts over the next fifteen years helped introduce Western treatment ideas, including the isolation of tuberculosis patients, a high-protein diet, and fundraising through the sale of Christmas seals to Korean Christians. But Hall was never able to treat more than a small number of patients, too few to have made a difference in overall mortality.[39]

In 1912 about 20 percent of boys and 1 percent of girls were enrolled in primary schools. Those proportions increased slowly through the 1920s, and then rapidly in the 1930s so that by 1940, 70 percent of boys and about 23 percent of girls were enrolled. Colonial authorities built more schools and trained more teachers. They also managed to raise the proportion of students attending school, but they did not expand the school system fast enough to keep up with demand. At primary school children studied a Japanese curriculum, usually in Japanese.[40]

Korean life expectancy rose from about 23.5 years during 1906–10 to about 42.6 years during 1936–40 and 44.9 years in 1942. Then began the years of turmoil, crisis, and devastation: from 1943 to 1945, in the latter stages of Japanese occupation; from 1945 to 1948, under Soviet and U.S. occupation of different parts of the country; and from 1950 to 1953, during the Korean War. Hae-Young Lee estimates South Korean casualties (i.e., deaths) during the war at 1.6 million.[41]

Once the war ended, life expectancy in South Korea surged, rising by six to eight years between the initial postwar estimates and 1960, even though there was as yet little economic development and little improvement in the standard of living. (Rapid economic growth began around 1964.)[42] Tai-Hwan Kwon and others attribute these gains to the introduction of antibiotics during the war and their widespread use after the war, an interpretation not entirely supported by the cause-of-death information assembled by E-Hyock Kwon and Tae-Ryong Kim.[43] Since such gains often occur after crises, some of the added years of survival may be a product of the restoration of conditions that had existed in the early 1940s.

Other factors may also have contributed. In 1947 U.S. authorities distributed Japanese assets seized at the end of the war, including land, industries, mines, and buildings, and in 1949 larger farms owned by Koreans were also seized for redistribution with fractional compensation.[44] Massive destruction of physical assets during the war also served to level Korean wealth. By the mid 1950s, wealth and income distribution had attained a degree of equitability unusual in a low-income country, and the traditional class system had been dismantled.[45] The earliest estimates for the distribution across households, for 1953 and the early 1960s, give Gini coefficients of 0.32 to 0.34.[46] That level was maintained into the 1970s, after which income distribution became more skew.[47] There was also rapid expansion in schooling in the earliest years after 1945, which inaugurated a period of several decades over which South Korea emerged as a world leader in the educational attainment of its populace.

The post–Korean War government invested heavily in social development, putting particular emphasis on education, health and welfare, and water supply, sanitation, and communications. That government also induced Koreans to spend much more than the government itself did on education, so that by the 1990s South Korea led the world in the proportion of GDP allotted to education at all levels.[48] Rapid gains in survival were revived for about twenty years after 1953, nearly matching the pace achieved between 1923 and 1937. A long period of poor to marginal nutrition, which had persisted since about 1910, narrowed in the 1960s when average daily calorie intake rose and people found access to a more diversified diet.[49] Fertility began to decline around 1960, while family planning programs helped reduce infant and child mortality.[50]

Conclusion

South Korea's most rapid gains in life expectancy preceded the period of its rapid gains in per capita income. The leading explanations for survival improvements in the Japanese era deal with certain aspects of social development, especially education, literacy, and school lessons in hygiene; and a wider provision of medical services. But those gains came amid immiseration of the Korean population, gauged by income and nutrition. The control of smallpox after 1920 contributed to better survival rates, as did also sanitary regulations introduced by the Japanese colonizers. Beginning in 1953 South Korea quickly recovered from a decade of devastation, surpassed the level of survival achieved by the early 1940s, and began to make rapid gains. Into the 1960s those rested once again on social development, including South Korea's emergence in the last part of the twentieth century as a world leader in the educational attainment of its people. The introduction of Western medicines and vaccines contributed to improvements in life expectancy, although those effects may have been spread over several years into the 1960s. Despite land reforms, which helped equalize the distribution of wealth and income, neither the government nor households could spend much more on health until the 1970s, when rapid economic growth led to higher discretionary spending by the government and by households. Poor nutrition remained a serious problem until the 1960s or 1970s. In sum, social growth played a more important role than economic growth at least until the 1960s, and was assisted by Japanese colonization, which laid the foundations of public health in Korea and built a medical system as well. The period 1943–53 interrupted Korea's gains and bifurcated the land between South and North, although both parts of the peninsula appear to have recovered the prewar survival position quickly after 1953.

Periods of rising inequality in the distribution of income, in Japan from the 1890s to the 1920s or Korea from 1970 to 1985, did not prevent survival gains. But in general a low level of income inequality has coincided with survival gains in Japan and South Korea.

The leading factors in Japan's attainment of a position of high life expectancy before it became a rich country begin with the control of cholera by quarantine and smallpox by vaccination in the last part of the nineteenth century. At the same time Japan also began to build a Western-style medical system, albeit one in which physicians were more numerous rather than highly specialized in their training. Unusually rapid progress in survival came during the 1910s and most of the 1920s, amid impressive gains in schooling that included the proportion of girls with primary schooling matching that of boys by 1911. The government's decision to shift resources toward militarization slowed that progress. During the 1930s the Japanese people, depending on their own resources, continued to make slow gains despite the heavy cost of tuberculosis and the government's hostile actions.

After World War II the Japanese quickly brought tuberculosis and typhoid fever under control, reduced infant and childhood mortality, and began a lengthy and successful campaign against cardiovascular disease. The result was a quick recovery of prewar life expectancy and extraordinarily rapid progress, to the point in 1978 of becoming the world's leader in survival. In Japan as in South Korea social growth led the way toward high life expectancy, and economic growth contributed only later.

CHAPTER 4

Very Low Income
Is Not a Barrier

Sri Lanka

The colonization of a country has often impeded social as well as economic development, and Ceylon / Sri Lanka has had an exceptionally long history of colonization under the Portuguese (1505 to 1658), the Dutch (to 1795), and the British (to 1948). In many of its colonies Britain imposed trading rules that stymied local economic development. Even though British investment often built a plantation sector and led to sharply increased exports of primary goods (in Ceylon's case especially coffee), few of the profits from trade worked their way into the pockets or the standard of living of the local population. Ceylon is an exception, however, not because economic development made much headway there, but because at least as early as the 1910s and 1920s the local population seized opportunities for social development. Local demand for health care, schools, and other social amenities remained strong after independence in 1948, and persisted after the economic reforms of 1977 that reoriented economic policy toward capitalism and private sector development and targeted only the lowest income groups for food subsidies.

During the 1990s increasing violence associated with the demands of the Tamil ethnic group for autonomy led to higher military spending at the cost of social programs, but authorities maintain that life expectancy gains continued or even quickened. Throughout, Sri Lanka's life expectancy gains have been achieved despite its continuing position as a country with a low level of per capita income, even among its low-income peer countries, and unusually high levels of undernutrition among infants and children.

Tracking Changes in Sri Lanka

Sri Lanka passed from Dutch to British administration at the beginning of 1796. At different points in the nineteenth century British colonial authorities introduced public health and medical institutions and innovations, including a training facility for physicians in 1870, hospitals for soldiers and later for civilians, a system for registering births and deaths, smallpox vaccination, and some regulation of the living conditions of indentured Tamil Indian laborers working on plantations. While the effect of these reforms, and of efforts at cholera control in the 1880s and 1890s, may have been positive, they do not appear to have inaugurated the persistent decline in mortality associated with a health transition. For Sri Lanka, that transition did not begin until the early 1920s.[1]

Most scholarly authorities track the official crude death rates (deaths per 1,000 in the population), but because the reporting of deaths was incomplete, those understate mortality. Making rough corrections, a United Nations team concluded that Sri Lanka's crude death rate probably averaged between 38 and 42 in the period 1871–1910, or 10 to 20 deaths per 1,000 higher than official estimates.[2] Various authorities have estimated life expectancy from the first years of the twentieth century forward and Figure 12 shows an averaging of these sources' data. Values for 1901, 1911, and 1921 rely on official data, and therefore probably overstate life expectancy, but after that time the estimates are very similar for each year, which adds some confidence to their reliability and accuracy.[3]

Figure 13 selects my preferred estimates in order to show the pace of gains in survival between each pair of estimates.[4] Three periods of improvement can be distinguished:

1. From the early 1920s to 1941, with the most rapid gains in life expectancy preceding the serious 1934–35 malaria epidemic.[5] Food shortages, caused by the loss of access to Japanese-occupied Burma, and higher malaria mortality made the war years and 1945–46 a time of high mortality;

2. From 1947 to 1953 or 1954, with almost unprecedentedly rapid gains in survival despite year-to-year variations;

3. From 1954 to 2000, a period of sustained gains at a slower pace, but ending with more robust gains in the late 1990s despite the high level of life expectancy already achieved.[6]

And figure 14 shows these preferred estimates of life expectancy together with Maddison's estimates of GDPpc.[7] In the nineteenth century income

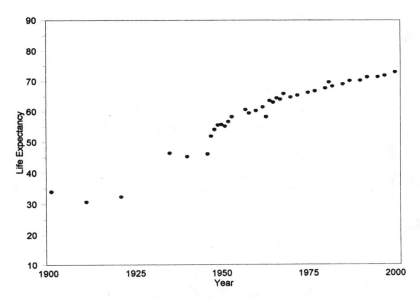

FIGURE 12. Life expectancy estimates for Sri Lanka, 1901–2000.
SOURCE: James C. Riley, "Bibliography of Works Providing Estimates of
Life Expectancy at Birth and of the Beginning Period of Health Transitions
in Countries with a Population in 2000 of at least 400,000" at www.lifetable
.de/RileyBib.htm.

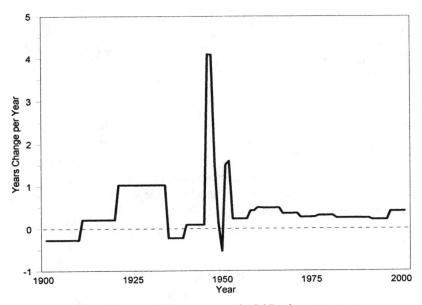

FIGURE 13. Pace of change in life expectancy in Sri Lanka, 1901–2000.
SOURCE: James C. Riley, "Bibliography of Works Providing Estimates of
Life Expectancy at Birth and of the Beginning Period of Health Transitions
in Countries with a Population in 2000 of at least 400,000" at www.lifetable
.de/RileyBib.htm.

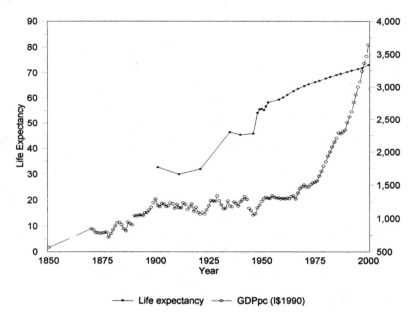

FIGURE 14. Life expectancy and gross domestic product per capita (GDPpc) in 1990 international dollars (I$) in Sri Lanka, 1850–2000.
SOURCES: Angus Maddison, *The World Economy: Historical Statistics* (Paris: Development Center of the Organization for Economic Cooperation and Development, 2003), pp. 181–85; and James C. Riley, "Bibliography of Works Providing Estimates of Life Expectancy at Birth and of the Beginning Period of Health Transitions in Countries with a Population in 2000 of at least 400,000" at www.lifetable.de/RileyBib.htm.

gains occurred without improvements in survival; the higher income may have been claimed mostly by plantation owners. The I$ 1,000 plateau was passed around 1890. In the period 1920–54, gains in life expectancy occurred without gains in income per capita; a wartime shrinkage in income was followed by recovery only to the previous level. Since the late 1960s, and especially since 1977, however, gains in income have been rapid and substantial. Sri Lanka's position as a low-income country with high life expectancy was attained by the end of the period 1921–54, during which GDPpc averaged about I$ 1,200 and deviated little from that figure, while life expectancy passed 60 in 1960. There is no indication that gains in per capita income played a part in improving survival, but the country's status as a land that could afford to invest in medicine, education, and public health was important.

Health Initiatives

Although vital statistics and cause-of-death data were collected imper-
fectly, there is a particularly rich body of information about health initiatives in British Sri Lanka, with the initiatives often being described in
convincing detail. Table 9 assembles explanations for survival gains in the
period from the 1920s to 1941, and table 10 treats the years just after World
War II. Three areas stand out. First, significant public health improvements began in the 1910s, when a campaign against hookworm (a parasite that causes enervation and anemia) sought to persuade householders
to add latrines.[8] In later years new initiatives appeared, some overlapping
with improvements in the health care system, among which the health
centers (called health units) providing maternal and infant child care seem
to have been particularly effective. Funded by government investments
rather than by patients and users, these centers drew more people into re-
ceiving health services, and the number of centers rose quickly in the 1930s.
Margaret Jones reports that these services developed over time between
the 1920s and 1948 and were generally available by 1948.[9]

Second, in the 1930s and 1940s colonial Sri Lanka began to construct
what Godfrey Gunatilleke terms a "welfare system" and others call a system of state socialism. The main elements of this system were free education; free health care for pregnant women, infants and young children;
and school meals and food subsidies.[10] Universal adult suffrage was introduced in Ceylon in 1931, along with competitive party politics and local control of domestic policies, which created a politically engaged elec-
torate that supported these programs.[11] From the late 1930s, when school
meals began to be served, the public sector also began to pay for nutritional supplements for children. Those programs faltered during World
War II, but were revived and extended into new areas after the war. By
1948, when Ceylon gained independence, most elements of this system
were in place. Thus British colonial control did not prevent local initiatives that democratized access to health care, foods, and schooling. Key
steps toward a welfare pattern of social development were taken in the
1910s, 1920s, and 1930s, both before and after the major political reforms
of 1931. Some measures, especially in the education of religious leaders,
developed from much older roots, predating Portuguese influence, and
from the late nineteenth-century Buddhist Reform Movement and its
teachings about health and healthy behaviors.[12]

Although not enough research has yet been done on the content of
school texts and adult education materials to establish how schooling may
have influenced health, literacy was evidently rising in every cohort from

TABLE 9. Explanations for Survival Gains in Sri Lanka from the Early 1920s to 1941

Area	Innovations	Leading Effects
Public health	Sanitation branch was added to medical department in 1913, more active after World War I	
	Rockefeller Foundation campaign against hookworm began 1916	1. People stopped defecating in the bush and used latrines, reducing fecal disease
		2. Prevalence and gravity of hookworm infestation was reduced
		3. Campaign may have alleviated co-morbidities, especially tuberculosis
	Smallpox vaccinations continued apace (from the 1890s), and more typhoid fever vaccinations were made	Smallpox remained infrequent, and fecal disease was further reduced
	Public health activity was curtailed by the economic depression of the 1930's.	Curtailed activity did not result in any apparent slowdown in survival gain.
Medicine and individual behavior	Hospitals were supplemented by health units and a sharply rising number of health centers	1. The health units promoted maternal and infant health, health education, sanitation, and school health work, but provided treatment only for hookworm
		2. Health centers increased from 40 in 1930 to 408 in 1939, accompanied by more visits by pregnant women and infants/children
	Medical exams of school children were instituted	Earlier/better detection of some problems, especially hookworm, resulted
	More midwives were trained	Safer childbirths resulted

the 1890s forward in time, and faster for females, who initially lagged well behind males.[13] Figure 15 shows the results of Sri Lanka's 1971 census questions on literacy, reported by age and sex. Females seem to have benefited more than males from the implementation of free education in 1944, which led to a sharper rise in literacy for the cohort born in the later 1930s. But there are no other signs of particular unevenness in literacy gains.

TABLE 9. (*continued*)

Area	Innovations	Leading Effects
Education	More schools opened, more children, especially males, received primary schooling	More people were prepared to understand contents of health education
Economic progress	Irrigation was expanded, and new roads and railroads were built	Fewer and less severe food shortages resulted, up to 1941

SOURCES: Dallas F. S. Fernando, "Health Statistics in Sri Lanka, 1921–80," in *Good Health at Low Cost,* ed. Scott B. Halstead, Julia A. Walsh, and Kenneth S. Warren (New York: Rockefeller Foundation, 1985), pp. 79–92; Godfrey Gunatilleke, "Health and Development in Sri Lanka—An Overview," in *Good Health at Low Cost,* pp. 111–24; Gunatilleke, "Sri Lanka's Social Achievements and Challenges," in *Social Development and Public Policy: A Study of Some Successful Experiences,* ed. Dharam Ghai (New York: St. Martin's, 2000), pp. 139–52; Christopher Langford, "Reasons for the Decline in Mortality in Sri Lanka Immediately after the Second World War: A Re-examination of the Evidence," *Health Transition Review* 6 (1996): 3–23; Srinivasa A. Meegama, "The Decline of Mortality in Sri Lanka in Historical Perspective," *International Population Conference Manila 1981,* 3 vols. (Liège: International Union for the Scientific Study of Population, 1981), 2: 143–64; and United Nations, Economic and Social Commission for Asia and the Pacific, *Population of Sri Lanka* (Bangkok: ESCAP, 1976), pp. 123–53, 208–22.

A great deal of attention has been and continues to be given to the third health innovation, the program of mosquito control begun in November 1945 with the spraying of DDT, an insecticide nearly insoluble in water that persisted in the environment much longer than the other insecticides then available. This characteristic made DDT more effective for mosquito control than the main insecticide previously used, Paris green (but DDT was also later found to threaten other insects and organisms up the food chain). Survival gains were rapid in the next few years. Estimates of the proportion of those gains attributable to mosquito control range from under 16 percent to over 40 percent. Even though extensive information is available, the statistical data—chiefly crude death rates and cause-of-death statistics assigning most deaths to symptoms rather than to specific diseases—are inadequate to fix the precise level of DDT's impact.[14] Official cause-of-death statistics, which are incomplete, suggest that malaria mortality dropped from 820 deaths per million in 1938 to 206 in 1951 and 0.1 in 1958, before beginning to rise again in 1968.[15] But several authorities have argued that mortality also declined sharply in areas with little incidence of the disease as well as in malaria areas. In the end it seems likely that mosquito control played a large but not a determining role in the postwar portion of Sri Lanka's mortality decline. Malaria mortality

TABLE 10. Explanations for Survival Gains in Sri Lanka, 1946–1954

Area	Innovations	Leading Effects
Public health	Mosquito control via DDT was initiated November 1945	Population of anopheles vectors of malaria was reduced, hence also incidence of malaria
	Prewar public health activity revived	Mortality resumed its prewar downward trend
	New vaccines were introduced	Adding protection against new diseases to the existing smallpox and typhoid fever vaccinations prevented many diseases
Medicine	Number of health centers rose from 437 in 1942 to 744 in 1954	Maternal and infant mortality declined
	Antibiotics were introduced.	Antibiotics reduced mortality in many bacterial diseases
Nutrition	Wartime shortages ended; school meals program expanded; free milk distributed	Infant and child nutrition improved; hence poor nutrition, a factor especially in the outcome of sicknesses, was reduced
	The government funded food subsidies	Subsidies reduced undernutrition for all age groups
Education	Free schooling at all levels was instituted in 1944	Males still led in literacy, but levels for the entire population improved
Economic progress	Welfare system was created	Mortality risks faced by poorest segments of populace were reduced

SOURCES: Dallas F. S. Fernando, "Health Statistics in Sri Lanka, 1921–80," in *Good Health at Low Cost,* ed. Scott B. Halstead, Julia A. Walsh, and Kenneth S. Warren (New York: Rockefeller Foundation, 1985), pp. 79–92; Godfrey Gunatilleke, "Health and Development in Sri Lanka—An Overview," in *Good Health at Low Cost,* pp. 111–24; Gunatilleke, "Sri Lanka's Social Achievements and Challenges," in *Social Development and Public Policy: A Study of Some Successful Experiences,* ed. Dharam Ghai (New York: St. John's, 2000), pp. 139–52; Christopher Langford, "Reasons for the Decline in Mortality in Sri Lanka Immediately after the Second World War: A Re-examination of the Evidence," *Health Transition Review* 6 (1996): 3–23; Srinivasa A. Meegama, "The Decline of Mortality in Sri Lanka in Historical Perspective," *International Population Conference Manila 1981,* 3 vols. (Liège: International Union for the Scientific Study of Population, 1981), 2: 143–64; and United Nations, Economic and Social Commission for Asia and the Pacific, *Population of Sri Lanka* (Bangkok: ESCAP, 1976), pp. 123–53, 208–22.

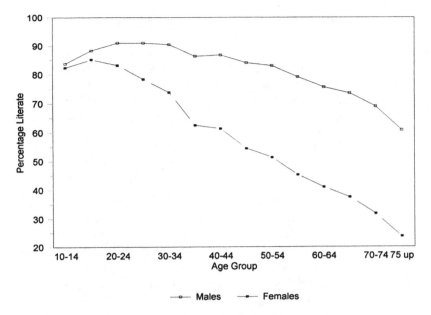

FIGURE 15. Literacy in Sri Lanka in 1971 by age and sex.
SOURCE: *Adult Literacy in Sri Lanka: A Survey of Literacy among the Adult Population in Eight Districts of Sri Lanka*, 2 vols. (Colombo: National Association for Total Education, 1990), 1: 6.

was high in the 1930s, even excluding the epidemic of 1934–35; it was very low by the mid 1950s and remained low into the 1970s; the main explanation available to account for this decline is mosquito control using DDT.

If one explanation of Sri Lanka's health transition argues that public health innovations led to most of the mortality decline, and a second that DDT-spraying was the largest single factor in the years when gains were most dramatic, later developments underscore the importance of continuing expansion in the country's welfare system.[16] Maternal mortality fell especially after 1947, assisted by malaria control but also by the introduction of family planning in 1953.[17] In the third period of Sri Lankan survival gains, from 1954 to the present, mortality continued to decline despite the reemergence of malaria in 1968 and despite the long economic malaise of 1961–77, which led some authorities, especially Srinivasa Meegama, to worry that progress would cease.[18] The number of health centers, physicians, nurses, hospital beds, and other indices of the availability of health care rose from the 1960s, although not all of them as rapidly as the population increased.[19] Mortality among adults and older adults declined. The transition from economic malaise to growth around 1977 does not appear, from World Bank estimates of life expectancy, to have led quickly to more rapid gains in survival. After 1977 the welfare system remained in place and contributed in an important way to continuing gains, which Sri Lanka was able to make despite "the persistence of poverty, malnutrition and unemployment" and Tamil unrest.[20]

Conclusion

Higher quality age-specific cause-of-death statistics might make it possible to allocate responsibility more firmly among the explanations offered for survival gains in Sri Lanka. But the timing of gains and of interventions makes it apparent that each stage of intervention brought noteworthy improvement and that each stage played a significant role in the country's transition from a low- to a high-survivorship community. Public health innovations made in the 1920s and 1930s, Sri Lanka's welfare system, and DDT-spraying in the period 1945–53 have been the leading factors cited to explain this country's achievement of high life expectancy. But the welfare system was still in the early stages of construction when Sri Lanka's health transition began, in the 1920s, and during the period of most rapid gains in survival up to 1945. Thus it is more convincing to cite state socialism as a factor in survival gains after 1945 than before. Up to 1945 the most important factors in reducing mortality seem to have been the wider provision of health care, especially to infants and mothers, through health centers; a pattern of rising educational attainment (aided by free tuition from 1944) in which girls caught up with boys; more individual responsibility for safely managing the disposal of human waste; and nutritional supplements for school children and food subsidies for the general population.

CHAPTER 5

Two Neighbors

Panama and Costa Rica

The neighboring countries Panama and Costa Rica share some important similarities. At first glance their life expectancy histories also appear to be similar. Both initiated health transitions in the period from the 1890s to the 1910s, and both matched the rich lands in achieving high life expectancy by the 1950s. But the history behind those health transitions, and the ways in which high survival was attained, could hardly contrast more starkly.

Panama

Panama's development was much affected by its connection with the United States. In the first years of the twentieth century, the United States took over the abandoned French project to build a canal across the Isthmus of Panama, fostered Panama's independence from Columbia in 1903, and quickly negotiated the lease of the 10-mile wide Canal Zone from the new nation. Organizing for construction began in 1904, and the canal was completed 1914. The French project of 1879–89 had included little activity toward controlling yellow fever, malaria, and other diseases, and many canal laborers and supervisors had died. The U.S. project, by contrast, began with a disease control program, although one not initially supported by the military commander in charge. Most elements of the program were copied from the public health efforts of U.S. authorities in Havana in 1899–1902, where yellow fever and malaria had been brought under control in the aftermath of the Spanish-American War. In Panama, as in Havana, the program began with an assault on yellow fever and *Aedes aegypti,* a mosquito vector that prefers to live in and around human dwellings, and then was expanded to include malaria and its anopheles mosquito vectors, as well as houseflies and other pests. One blood-parasite survey suggested that up to 80 percent of the indigenous population in the 47-mile-long band where the canal was to be built was infected with malaria.

U.S. health workers in Panama called their approach the Gorgas method, after William C. Gorgas, who had led the effort in Cuba and who directed public health activities in the area of canal building in Panama from 1904 to 1914. Gorgas's method had three key elements. First, Gorgas decided to focus disease-control activities not just on the U.S.-controlled Canal Zone, but on the cities and villages within that zone, especially settled sites within a mile of the canal on either side, and he attempted to segregate the populations inside that space from those outside. Even though the Panama Canal health department by 1912 had 1,373 employees and "an army of inspectors," these labor-intensive measures could not have been extended to the entire country or even to the entire zone. Up to 1914, and to some degree beyond that year, activity remained concentrated in about 100 square miles of the 500-square mile zone. (Panama has some 29,000 square miles.)

The second part of the Gorgas method was a broad attack on mosquitoes. Sanitary inspectors visited homes to point out mosquito-breeding sites inside and outside; fumigated with sulfur or pyrethrum; installed wire screens; removed people suffering from yellow fever to isolation hospitals; hired mosquito catchers; and instructed people about how to use chloroform in test tubes to kill mosquitoes resting on walls. The U.S. team set about to clear the brush, drain standing water, and build permanent drainage ditches, also within this two mile wide band. Where necessary, inspectors also supervised the preparation and use of crude oil and heated oil sprays as larvicides and, later, the introduction of larvae-eating fish at anopheles breeding sites.

Third, the Gorgas approach devised means of enforcement, relying on discipline and, for Panamanians in the canal-building area, behavior modification. Members of the U.S. military, who had the authority to order subordinates and civilian employees to follow directions, directed the project and its associated public health program. For Panamanians, who could not be ordered around as easily, Gorgas and his associates levied fines well beyond most people's ability to pay, then withdrew the fine when people obeyed orders. Regular visits to houses gave sanitary inspectors the information they needed to detect violations, assess fines, and decide whether to release people from fines.[1]

In Panama City, Colon, and Canal Zone housing camps the Americans also introduced the filtration and chlorination of water, connecting most houses to the water system and to a parallel system for removing and treating human waste. And they controlled other disease vectors, including houseflies. The concession of the Canal Zone to the United States brought Panama an initial sum of money plus an annual payment of $2 million, resources that were used in part for social projects in Panama City and Colon over and above what U.S. authorities invested there.

These activities had the desired effect in the two-mile band along the canal for Panamanians, laborers from Jamaica, Barbados, Italy, and elsewhere, and Americans.[2] The mosquito control program reduced mortality from yellow fever and malaria and days missed from work on the canal owing to malaria to a small fraction of the initial level. The water and sewage treatment programs suppressed both mortality and sickness from typhoid fever and dysentery. Among employees mortality and sickness, or morbidity, plunged between 1906 and 1916 and remained low. In the portion of the Canal Zone from which statistics were collected, mortality declined a few years earlier and more sharply than in Panama City and Colon, but there, too, these improvements had a strong and beneficent effect.[3]

But the improvements did little or nothing for the rest of the country.[4] Construction of the canal divided Panama into two parts. The area of the Canal Zone and the contiguous cities of Panama and Colon moved quickly into the status of a low mortality region. But the "interior" benefited little, given the U.S. policy that "it is impractical to attempt to sanitate the country" or even to do more for Panamanian laborers who cleared land and built drainage ditches than to give them quinine.[5] Although *interioranos* sometimes moved into and out of the zone, they were not allowed within one mile of army posts and residential areas of the two-mile band and for the most part remained isolated from the economic, social, and public health activities of the canal area. This division was still in place in the 1950s, when John and Mavis Biesanz examined race, class, and living conditions in Panama—with one exception that amounted to a step backwards: the urban poor of Panama City and Colon in the 1950s resembled the *interioranos* in health more than they did the employees of the Canal Zone and their family members.[6]

Even though only a small fraction of the populace lived in the areas

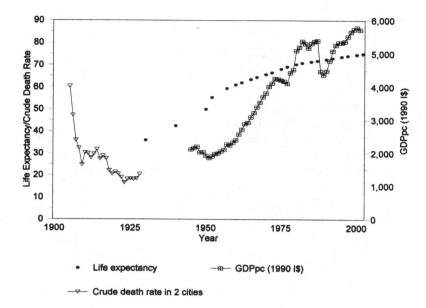

FIGURE 16. Life expectancy, crude death rates, and gross domestic product per capita (GDPc) in 1990 international dollars (I$) in Panama, 1905–2000. SOURCES: Angus Maddison, *The World Economy: Historical Statistics* (Paris: Development Center of the Organization for Economic Cooperation and Development, 2003), pp. 146, 148; and James C. Riley, "Bibliography of Works Providing Estimates of Life Expectancy at Birth and of the Beginning Period of Health Transitions in Countries with a Population in 2000 of at least 400,000" at www.lifetable.de/RileyBib.htm.

that benefited from public health improvements, the benefits they enjoyed seem to have been pronounced enough to have reduced the crude death rate in the main cities almost immediately and elevated life expectancy in the country as a whole as early as the 1920s. But early statistics on the *interioranos* are so meager that life expectancy gains reported for the country as a whole for the period 1904–40 (figure 16) may be misleading.[7]

Economic development was similarly bifurcated. The development that accompanied canal use was concentrated chiefly in Panama City and Colon, which gained a much higher standard of living than did the agricultural hinterlands. By about 1950 even the more impoverished segments of the urban population enjoyed better health facilities and opportunities for schooling than *interioranos*. Deaths in cities were much likelier to be attended by trained medical providers, and death rates there were lower.

By 1971 slightly more than two-fifths of the country's people lived in the advantaged area around the Canal Zone or in the zone, versus about a third in 1940 and about a quarter in 1920.

A 1904 law obliged the government to provide schools and teachers for students aged 7–15, and literacy rose between the censuses of 1911 and 1950. But Robert Looney reports that, as of 1975, only about a third of children in this age group attended school, even though government spending on education, as on health, was unusually high compared to other Latin American countries and even though many new schools had been opened in rural areas. Attendance rates did not begin to rise until the late 1960s.[8]

Estimates of life expectancy from Panamanian sources, the United Nations, and the World Bank all suggest that by the 1950s Panama had achieved the status of a poor country with high life expectancy. But descriptive information about the standard of living and the disease burden of *interioranos* calls this into question. It seems likelier that life expectancy resembled that of the rich countries only in the area of the canal plus Panama City and Colon, where also the standard of living was higher than suggested by Maddison's estimates of GDPpc in figure 16. Thus Panama may not actually fit the bill as a country with better health than its income level would seem to warrant.

Costa Rica

Because some churches recorded baptisms, marriages, and burials from early colonial times, Costa Rica has an unusually long and rich mortality record—one of the many ways it differs from Panama. Figure 17 shows several estimates of life expectancy beginning with the 1860s, as well as Héctor Pérez Brignoli's reconstruction from the 1750s to the 1950s, which is based on crude death rates from population samples and certain assumptions about the age pattern of mortality. Pérez Brignoli suggests that life expectancy in that period varied between 21.4 and 46.1 years, but did not show a sustained pattern of improvement until the 1920s and did not exceed 46.1 until the late 1940s. Other estimates, made by Luis Rosero Bixby, indicate that sustained gains began earlier.[9] There is also uncertainty about the level of life expectancy in the 1870s and 1880s, which Pérez Brignoli estimates to have been above 35 years but Rosero Bixby places under 30. If Pérez Brignoli is correct, then Costa Rica's health transition began in the 1920s. But if Rosero Bixby is correct, it began earlier, perhaps in

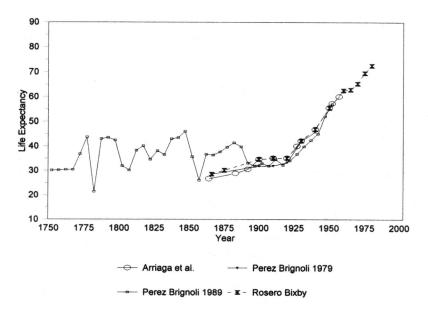

—○— Arriaga et al.   —•— Perez Brignoli 1979

—•— Perez Brignoli 1989   - **x** - Rosero Bixby

FIGURE 17. Life expectancy estimates for Costa Rica, 1750–2000.
SOURCES: Eduardo E. Arriaga, *New Life Tables for Latin American Populations
in the Nineteenth and Twentieth Centuries* (Berkeley: University of California
Press, 1968), pp. 82–91, 98–99; Héctor Pérez Brignoli, "Notas sobre el descenso de la mortalidad en Costa Rica (1866–1973)," in *Sétimo seminario naciónal
de demografía* (San José: n.p., 1979), pp. 44–56; Pérez Brignoli, *El crecimiento
demográfico de America Latina en los siglos XIX y XX: Problemas, metodos y perspectives* (San Jose: Centro de Investigaciones Historicas, Universidad de Costa
Rica, 1989), p. 12; and Luis Rosero Bixby, "Determinantes del descenso de la
mortalidad infantil en Costa Rica," in *Demografía y epidemiología en Costa Rica*
(San José: Asociación Demográfica Costarricense, 1985), pp. 9–36.

the 1890s. Choosing between the interpretations requires more evidence
than is now available, but my inclination is to favor the 1890s as a beginning period.[10]

Figure 18 adds Maddison's GDPpc estimates from 1920. Income (in
constant 1990 values) averaged I\$ 1,650 in the 1920s and did not begin to
grow until the late 1940s. Clearly the 1920s level represents a certain degree of development, surpassing other Central American states except for
Panama, and suggests prior growth that needs to be situated chronolog-
ically because it may have contributed to gains in survival. If life expectancy
gains began as late as the 1920s, then Costa Rica fits in the middle of income levels achieved by states that began health transitions in the nineteenth century and cannot be considered precocious.

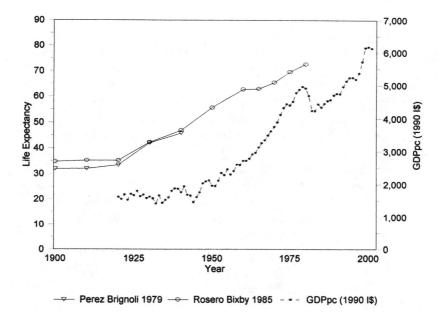

FIGURE 18. Life expectancy and gross domestic product per capita (GDPpc) in 1990 international dollars (I$) in Costa Rica, 1750–2000.
SOURCES: Héctor Pérez Brignoli, "Notas sobre el descenso de la mortalidad en Costa Rica (1866–1973)," in *Sétimo seminario naciónal de demografía* (San José: n.p., 1979), pp. 44–56; Angus Maddison, *The World Economy: Historical Statistics* (Paris: Development Center of the Organization for Economic Cooperation and Development, 2003), pp. 145–47; and Luis Rosero Bixby, "Determinantes del descenso de la mortalidad infantil en Costa Rica," in *Demografía y epidemiología en Costa Rica* (San José: Asociación Demográfica Costarricense, 1985), pp. 9–36.

The years from the 1870s to 1920 saw important economic changes in Costa Rica. Plantation agriculture expanded, with coffee exports rising from the 1850s up to the early 1900s. The completion of a railroad from the capital of San José to the Atlantic coast in 1890 allowed coffee sales to Great Britain to grow more rapidly, after about fifty years of slow expansion. Banana exports grew from 111,000 bunches in 1883 to a peak of 11.2 million bunches in 1913. While coffee was cultivated in the central highlands, near San José, bananas were grown on the Atlantic coast, a malaria zone. Thus, banana exports meant high mortality for the mostly immigrant population that worked the banana plantations. Most of those laborers came from Jamaica, and the literature leaves unclear whether their numbers and deaths have been included in national estimates.[11]

Scholars who have examined Costa Rica's health transition have some disagreements about the specific factors that contributed to it, but agree that this was a transition with multiple causes, none of dominant strength. Also, as figure 17 showed, the approximate pace of change in life expectancy before the 1920s was slow and the gains meager.

Although it was not until the administration of the physician Rafael Calderón as president (1940–44) that Costa Rica adopted policies intended to fully share the rewards of economic growth with lower income groups, important features of social development are evident from an earlier period. Between the censuses of 1891 and 1927, amid a program attempting to provide universal primary school education, reported literacy improved from 28 to 66 percent. New normal schools formed in the late nineteenth century trained waves of mostly female teachers, some from rural and artisanal backgrounds and some from the developing middle class of San José. As a result, by the 1890s women were in charge of the primary schools of the country. Hygiene was added to the normal school curriculum, and investments in schools and health facilities grew from the 1910s. (A strong communist party, which formed in 1931 and was especially active in banana-growing regions, also promoted health investments.) Between the 1890s and the 1920s smallpox vaccination reached an ever-larger share of the population. Public authorities and the medical community built hospitals and organized the delivery of medical services (see below). San José was provided with filtered water.

There were some factors that worked to Costa Rica's disadvantage—agriculture outside the plantation sector was mostly at subsistence levels; communications within most of the country remained poor, even after completion of the railroad link between San José and the Atlantic coast; and there were rising numbers of landless laborers. But the innovations in public health and education, plus the advantages of a homogeneous populace and a mostly stable political system after 1889, tipped the balance in favor of comparatively low underlying mortality. Rapid gains in survival then began rather suddenly in the early 1920s, and the pace of gains remained high up to about 1982, by which time life expectancy at birth had reached nearly 74 years.[12]

Ana Cecilia Román Trigo's compilation of public spending in the period 1870–1948 makes it easy to detect changing priorities, and in particular to distinguish spending on social functions—education, public health, housing, and social security—from other categories.[13] Figure 19 charts this path, showing social development spending as a percentage of all government spending. In the late 1880s Costa Rica began to allocate more to

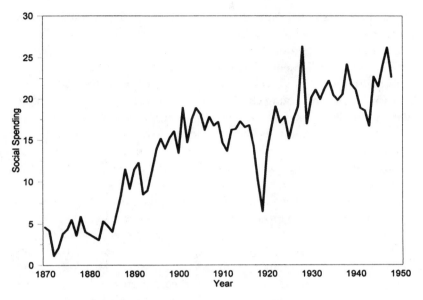

FIGURE 19. Social development spending as percentage of government
expenditures in Costa Rica, 1870–1948.
SOURCE: Ana Cecilia Román Trigo, *Las finanzas públicas de Costa Rica: Metodología y fuentes (1870–1948)* (San José: Centro de Investigaciones Históricas de
América Central, Universidad de Costa Rica, 1995), pp. 56–63.

primary education, and by 1900 social spending had jumped to nearly 14
percent of the total. That level was maintained into the 1920s before giving way, through the 1930s and 1940s, to another lengthy period of rising
social investment. By 1948 social spending approached 23 percent of total
spending. In that latter phase spending on education continued to grow,
but so did spending on public health and then social security.

Costa Rica began to build a modern health system in the 1890s, although here too progress was slow until the 1920s. An effective public
health system was begun in the 1910s and carried forward in the 1920s,
partly through local initiatives and partly through two outside initiatives:
the United Fruit Company's programs against hookworm and malaria
and the Rockefeller Foundation's campaign against hookworm and fecal
disease, which recruited allies among Costa Rica's women primary school
teachers. Malaria mortality among United Fruit Company employees declined in 1929 and following years, after the company began using the insecticide Paris green (copper acetoarsenate), draining camp sites, clean-

ing up breeding sites around living quarters, and giving workers the new drug Plasmochin, which was believed to kill malaria parasites in the sexual stage of their reproductive cycle.[14] Schools drilled students in lessons about health while the hookworm campaign reached many adults with information about why and how to build latrines. Preventive medical services for infants and young children were introduced in the 1920s, along with a campaign against tuberculosis in which health visitors sought to identify cases and counsel other people in the household about how to protect themselves from the disease. Although hard times in the 1930s brought retrenchment in new investments, survival continued to improve.

In 1942, following the election of Calderón as president, Costa Rica added health and maternity insurance, and in 1946 disability and old age pensions. From that period "the old oligarchic-liberal state evolved into a welfare (benefactor) state."[15] Many authorities have been sufficiently impressed with these innovations to suggest that the 1940s marked a watershed.[16] In fact, programs favoring social development had been emerging piece by piece since the 1890s. Thus the modern shift toward greater equality in the distribution of household income, which by 1971 put Costa Rica in the position of having one of the more egalitarian distributions in Latin America, occurred after the country achieved its status as a land of good health but low incomes.[17]

Antibiotics, effective against some fecal disease, which remained important causes of death, arrived in the late 1940s. Additionally, the United Fruit Company used DDT to control mosquitoes and malaria in an extensive spraying campaign of 1943–47, which coincided with the highest pace of gains in life expectancy ever attained in Costa Rica (figure 20; the 1920s also saw important gains with the beginnings of control of fecal disease). The supply of doctors, nurses, midwives, and hospital beds rose from the 1920s onward. The increasing share of deaths attended by physicians rather than lay practitioners, which grew from about 40 percent in 1927 to 60 percent in the late 1940s, suggests also that more people received formal medical attention. Primary school enrollments increased and literacy rose from 66 percent of the population aged 10 and up in 1927 to 79 percent in 1950 and 86 percent in 1963. By 1950 literacy among females surpassed that among males, which is a sign of female autonomy.[18]

Per capita income expanded again from the late 1940s, after decades of stagnation, and housing improved in many areas of the country. Up to that point Costa Rica's gains in survival were achieved despite stagnant economic indicators, and in the 1930s in the face of deteriorating conditions.

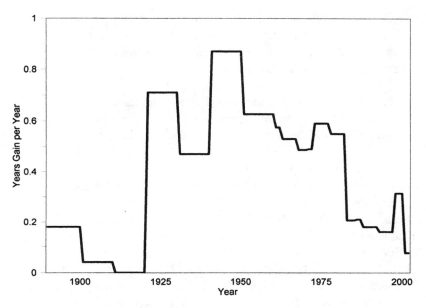

FIGURE 20. Pace of gains in life expectancy in Costa Rica, 1890–2000.
SOURCES: Leonardo Mata and Luis Rosero Bixby, *National Health and Social Development in Costa Rica: A Case Study of Intersectoral Action* (Washington: Pan American Health Organization, 1988), pp. 55–56; Luis Rosero Bixby, "Determinantes del descenso de la mortalidad infantil en Costa Rica," in *Demografía y epidemiología en Costa Rica* (San José: Asociación Demográfica Costarricense, 1985), pp. 9–36; and Luis Rosero Bixby and Herman Caamaño "Tablas de vida de Costa Rica, 1900–1980," in *Mortalidad y fecundidad en Costa Rica* (San José: Asociación Demográfica Costarricense, 1984), pp. 7–19.

San José had an appreciable advantage over the country as a whole in infant mortality by the early 1920s and widened that advantage in the decades that followed, up to the 1950s. Thus, a leading problem of the 1940s and 1950s was to bring rural areas up to the level of health in the capital. A Twentieth Century Fund team visited Costa Rica in 1950, and found that although San José's water and sanitation system may have needed repair and expansion, most rural areas still used water deemed unsafe to drink. Hookworm remained common in some locales, where many people defecated in cane fields or in the bush, habits associated with the spread of fecal disease. Nevertheless urbanization—the 19 percent of the population living in urban areas in 1927 rose to 29 percent in 1950— contributed something to survival gains, bringing more people into the ambit of urban health services.

Cause-of-death data affirm the importance of interventions that controlled fecal disease and malaria. Mortality from diarrhea and enteritis fell from 41.7 per 10,000 in 1931 to 18.7 in 1949, malaria mortality dropped dramatically during the DDT campaign, and tuberculosis mortality also declined.

Iván Molina Jiménez and Steven Palmer argue that Costa Rica began its path to becoming an interventionist state in the 1890s, with an orientation toward population health.[19] The most unusual feature of the Costa Rican system, compared to other low- and middle-income countries, is its expansive use of social insurance to pay for health care, some elements funded entirely by the public sector, others entirely by participants, and still others by contributions from both individuals and the state.[20] This health orientation withstood hard times in the 1930s and again in the 1980s, so that Costa Rica continued to converge toward the life expectancy achieved in high-income countries and, by 2002, had a life expectancy at birth of 77.6 years, which, according to UN estimates, surpassed the United States at 77.3 years. Another distinctive element for Costa Rica is that it disbanded its army in 1948, which has freed up significant resources for investment in other directions, including education and health.

Although there are no dominant factors in the history of mortality decline in Costa Rica, it is worth noting that (as figure 20 shows) two initiatives seem to have had a larger effect than any others: the control of fecal disease, which began in the 1920s and continued through the 1950s, and the control of malaria, which also began in the late 1920s and also continued into the 1950s.

Conclusion

Costa Rica began its health transition between the 1890s and the 1920s, but probably in the 1890s with its health investments, while Panama's transition began in the 1910s. Panama remained pretty consistently behind Costa Rica, although it was able from the 1920s to keep up with the pace of change set by its neighbor. But the paths followed contrasted starkly. Panama depended heavily on U.S. intervention, which aimed to make the territory of the Canal Zone safe enough for its citizens, who managed and administered canal construction and operation, and for the Panamanians and workers from around the Caribbean who labored on the canal. Direct U.S. involvement in the zone funded a sizable public health and sanitary apparatus with a disciplined approach to controlling mosquito-borne diseases using insecticides, larvicides, drainage, and, later, DDT, while U.S. subventions invested in health and education for Panamanians living in the zone and in Panama City and Colon underwrote the control of yellow fever, malaria, fecal disease, and tuberculosis, and the long-run improvement of survival in the zone. *Interioranos* did not fare so well, lagging in survival, access to schooling and health care, income, and in social development in general. Although official statistics suggest that Panama as a whole has a rich country's level of life expectancy, it seems necessary to wonder whether survival among *interioranos* and among the urban poor of Panama City and Colon has been and is measured as accurately as among people living close to the canal.

Costa Rica, in contrast, initiated and sustained its health transition almost exclusively on resources of its own, aided by a certain degree of development prior to the 1890s that was built mostly on coffee and banana exports. Molina Jiménez and Palmer describe this land as an interventionist state with an orientation toward population health, a status built piecemeal over time. The best-known elements in Costa Rica's social development were introduced in the 1940s in the form of social insurance and pensions and the formation of a welfare or benefactor state, but as this summary history shows, the institutions of social development—schools and general population literacy, health care facilities, and a population armed with information that helped people protect themselves from health risks—had been built beginning in the 1890s. Costa Ricans began to control malaria, fecal disease, and tuberculosis in campaigns begun in the 1910s and 1920s, decades before the availability of DDT or antibiotics. Investments in education began even earlier, in the late nineteenth century, and girls passed boys in years of schooling by 1950. Like Sri Lanka, Costa Rica has retained its commitment to social development despite changing political regimes and economic prospects.

CHAPTER 6

Capitalism and Communism, Dictatorship and Democracy

Cuba and Jamaica

Cuba and Jamaica are neighboring islands that have followed quite different political paths but have had similar life expectancy histories. With the
Spanish-American War of 1898 the United States took the former Spanish colony of Cuba into its sphere of influence. In fact, U.S. economic
influence on the island had been growing throughout the latter decades
of the nineteenth century, at Spain's expense, and would continue to grow
into the 1950s, well beyond the periods of U.S. occupation in 1898–1902,
1905–9, and 1917. Occupation brought direct intervention in Cuba's internal affairs, including public health, but the United States also inter-
fered in domestic policy during the years in between and from 1917 to
1959.

In 1953 a group of Cubans led by Fidel Castro launched a revolution
aimed at overthrowing the dictatorship of Fulgencio Batista; they succeeded in 1959. Castro then instituted Soviet-style economic and social
policies, shifting Cuba abruptly from capitalism dominated by outside
companies, mostly from the United States, to socialism dominated by Soviet ideals and assisted by Soviet economic support. That system persisted
to 1989, when the Soviet Union began to fall apart, but Castro has elected
to continue Soviet-style policies.

Jamaica had been a Spanish colony up to 1655, when the British took
over. Britain retained authority there until formal independence in 1962,
but from the 1890s, and especially from 1944, had turned a growing number of domestic matters over to Jamaicans. Nonetheless, the British practiced a kind of colonialist capitalism, maintaining open markets in Jamaica

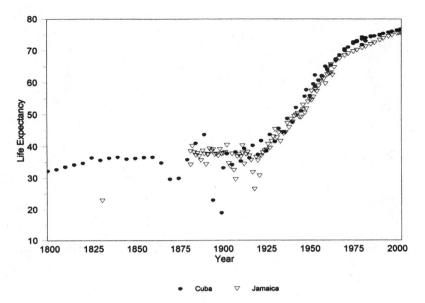

FIGURE 21. Life expectancy estimates for Cuba and Jamaica, 1800–2000.
SOURCES: James C. Riley, "Bibliography of Works Providing Estimates of
Life Expectancy at Birth and of the Beginning Period of Health Transitions
in Countries with a Population in 2000 of at least 400,000" at www.lifetable
.de/RileyBib.htm.

for British and Canadian interests, while limiting opportunities for Afro-
or Asian-Jamaicans to manufacture or trade in competition with British
or Canadian firms. Jamaica experimented briefly with the nationalization
of many firms and the creation of Cuban-style socialism under Michael
Manley in 1974 but in 1980, with the election of Edward Seaga, moved
back toward the open-market capitalism it had practiced in the 1950s and
1960s.

Figure 21 shows estimates of life expectancy in these two countries, for
Cuba from five sources and for Jamaica from three.[1] Both countries had
a similar level of life expectancy in the latter decades of the nineteenth century, at 36 to 38 years, with Jamaica slightly ahead. According to Rolando
Gonzalez Quiñones's estimates, Cuba pulled ahead in the early 1900s and
retained that advantage to the 1950s. In contrast estimates by Elio Velaz-
quez and Lázaro Toirac and by Alfonso Farnós Morejón suggest that
Cuba and Jamaica maintained much the same level and followed much
the same course from the 1920s to the 1950s, with Cuba keeping only a

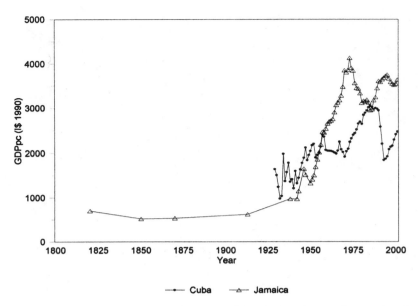

FIGURE 22. Gross domestic product per capita (GDPpc) in 1990 international dollars (I\$) in Cuba and Jamaica, 1820–2000.
SOURCE: Angus Maddison, *The World Economy: Historical Statistics* (Paris: Development Center of the Organization for Economic Cooperation and Development, 2003), pp. 145–48.

small advantage.[2] World Bank estimates from 1960, which are probably too high for Jamaica by about two years,[3] suggest that Cuba held an advantage by 1960, which it retained into the 1990s. In both countries the populace enjoyed rapidly improving survival prospects from the 1920s through the 1960s, with life expectancy rising from around 39 years in the 1920s in both countries to 68.4 years in Jamaica in 1970 and 70.3 years in Cuba. Thus it was within that period of about fifty years that Cuba and Jamaica distinguished themselves from most other low-income and low-survival countries.

Maddison supplies occasional estimates of GDPpc in 1990 international dollars for Jamaica before 1950 and annually thereafter; for Cuba he gives annual estimates from 1929 (see figure 22). Cuban sugar exports rose sharply but temporarily in the early 1890s, and again in the period 1902–25. One source estimates per capita income in Cuba in the 1922–25 period at more than 35 percent of the U.S. level, which, if accurate, would mean that GDPpc was higher then than in 1929.[4] Thus survival gains in the

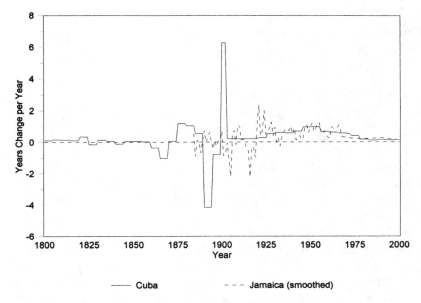

FIGURE 23. Pace of life expectancy change in Cuba and Jamaica, 1800–2000.
SOURCES: James C. Riley, "Bibliography of Works Providing Estimates of
Life Expectancy at Birth and of the Beginning Period of Health Transitions
in Countries with a Population in 2000 of at least 400,000" at www.lifetable
.de/RileyBib.htm.

early 1900s may have coincided with economic expansion in Cuba and
certainly coincided with larger sugar exports. But plantation economies
did not usually distribute income evenly across the population, and Cuba
is no exception.

From the 1920s to the end of World War II survival gains in Cuba and
Jamaica occurred with little or no improvement in per capita income. In
Jamaica income advanced rapidly in the 1950s and 1960s before falling back
in the 1970s and 1980s, while in Cuba per capita income peaked in 1959,
making the period 1945–59 the good years, followed by hard times that
lasted into the 1970s. There is little association between income gains or
losses and year-to-year changes in life expectancy, however. Cuba pulled
ahead of Jamaica in survival after 1960 despite having an economy that
generated a much lower standard of living as assessed by GDPpc.

As figure 23 shows, from the 1920s to 1970 both countries enjoyed not
just gains in survival but an unusually high pace of gains, with the pace
in Jamaica peaking in the 1920s and during 1945–55. Between 1945 and

1955 each country added years to life expectancy at a rate of just under 1 year gain per year of calendar time.

Cuba

Gonzalez Quiñones's estimates across the period 1799–1959 suggest that life expectancy gains in Cuba may have begun in the 1880s, after the unsuccessful war for independence of 1868–78, but were interrupted during the 1895–98 revolution against Spain and the Spanish-American War. Several authorities agree that life expectancy improved from around 1900, setting aside recovery from conditions in the 1890s, and that gains came at a slow pace until the 1920s. For the earlier period, up to the 1940s, Sergio Diaz Briquets and Garcia Quiñones stress a similar group of factors contributing to increased longevity: the sanitary policies introduced during the U.S. occupation of 1898–1902; economic growth, especially during 1905–24; rising rates of literacy and primary school enrollment in the period 1901–25; urbanization, which moved more of the population into locales with better health services; and the growing number of health facilities. Disparities in income within the Cuban populace were pronounced in the nineteenth century and remained so throughout the period 1900–1959. Thus it is not at all clear that economic growth translated into a higher standard of living for most people, especially for Cubans of African background. Although blacks made some gains in occupational mobility in the early decades of the twentieth century, those were reversed during the depression of the 1930s.[5]

Nevertheless the Cuban government earned higher tax revenues after 1900 and for some years spent significant amounts on public health, including sanitary services in Havana, smallpox vaccinations for the populace in general, and new hospitals. Cubans also developed a system of private health insurance provided through mutual societies, which gave working people access to medical care. These organizations appeared in the late nineteenth century and by the 1910s and 1920s enrolled a large share of the population.[6]

Walter Reed, William C. Gorgas, and other authorities from the United States set out in 1898 to control yellow fever, a worrisome mosquito-borne disease that they believed to be endemic in Cuba. Control of yellow fever in Cuba would, they hoped, help protect the United States. Thus they did not initially seek to suppress malaria, which was a more important cause of death and disability in Cuba itself. The U.S. public health team began with a house-to-house inspection of sanitary conditions, spraying mosquito breeding sites, and a program to persuade householders to cover water barrels outside their houses and containers inside. They soon added smallpox vaccinations. the isolation of people with tuberculosis in a new hospital (the leading U.S. measure of tuberculosis control), and the creation of an effective system of public health laws and administration.[7] Even though much of the literature on United States–Cuba relations emphasizes exploitation by the United States, nearly every commentator agrees that the cooperation between the health authorities of the two countries from 1899 to 1906 launched effective steps at controlling important diseases.

Cause-of-death statistics for Havana, with some 15 percent of the island's population in 1907, show that mortality from diseases associated with human waste and from tuberculosis, malaria, smallpox, and yellow fever declined, although in an irregular pattern.[8] Mortality from fecal disease was cut in half in the period 1901–7. Tuberculosis mortality dropped by about half between 1919 and 1931 and declined again between 1943 and 1953. Malaria mortality diminished in the early years of the century, as a collateral effect of the U.S.-led campaign against yellow fever, but also in a persistent way across the period 1910–50. There was some breakdown during the 1920s in the health programs the United States had fashioned in the early years of the century, but life expectancy gains continued nevertheless. Primary school enrollment peaked in 1925–26 at 63 percent of the school-age population and did not surpass that level again until the 1950s.[9] Across the period 1899–1931 black youths made much faster gains in literacy than did white counterparts, nearly closing the wide gap that had separated the two groups in 1899.[10]

After World War II the arrival of antibiotics and, during the 1950s, wider use of vaccines can be added to this list of disease control factors. Survival gains continued even though per capita spending on health services declined and disparities in income and access to health services by region, race, and income level remained in place.

The 1959 revolution brought fundamental political and socioeconomic changes. The ruling class was overturned, and with it longstanding bias against people of African background and against low-income groups. Many members of the elite, including about half the country's physicians, emigrated. The new government set out systematically to remove disparities in access to health care, training more providers, building new health and sanitation facilities in rural areas, even educating physicians about how to discuss health issues with those patients who had little or no schooling. Likewise the revolution brought a massive development of the educational system and a literacy campaign aimed at adults. In reaction to the revolution, the United States declared a trade embargo. This had little effect, however, until the collapse of the Soviet Union, which had provided subsidies for Cuba. Then, in the 1990s, the health system deteriorated as medications and supplies became more difficult to obtain.[11]

The emigration in 1959 of a substantial proportion of people with the highest incomes and best survival prospects might have brought an immediate reduction in life expectancy. But the revolution's health initiatives successfully attacked regional, racial, and class groups previously underserved.[12] Survival gains continued at a high pace through the 1960s (life expectancy in 1960 was already as high as 64 to 65 years). The revolution did not alter the course of life expectancy gains as life expectancy among blacks rose to near equality with whites.[13]

Economic development, income distribution, access to health and sanitation services, political stability, corruption, and the development of literacy and education had all been inconstant allies or opponents of survival gains in Cuba. The initiatives of the period 1900–1925 appear to have created a strong enough public health infrastructure to withstand the inconstancy of these factors in the period 1925–59. The Cuban case suggests that a strong beginning in the development of public health and, later, medical services may be enough to carry a country forward for many years of indifferent investment or even disinvestment. From that perspective there have been two long-run cycles of public sector engagement. The first ran from about 1900 to 1959, with public health services leading initially, and the period after about 1925 marked by disinvestments. The second ran from 1959 to 2005 with medical services leading, and the period after 1989 marked by disinvestments.[14]

Jamaica

Jamaica's health transition began rather abruptly in the 1920s and was led by sharp declines in mortality from malaria, tuberculosis, and diseases associated with human fecal matter, all leading causes of death. The foundations for disease control had been laid in the prior decades, in the expansion of the primary school system, which offered free schooling, a rapid rise in female enrollments, and the creation of an island medical corps that served rural areas as well as Kingston. By the 1910s Jamaicans were receptive to the idea that schooling brought rewards, if seldom the economic advancement they had hoped for. The school curriculum was widened in the 1910s to add hygiene education, initially for teachers-in-training and then for students.[15]

The Rockefeller Foundation's hookworm campaign team arrived in 1919 and found Jamaicans open to the idea of community engagement in public health and to a series of campaigns against specific diseases. The first campaign aimed to build latrines for homes and schools and to teach Jamaicans how and why to use them. By 1926 the basic hookworm campaign had evolved into a broad attack against the leading causes of death. Educational material was its main weapon: pithy and explicit advice about disease avoidance, accessible explanations about germs and disease vectors, and effective information about what individuals could do to protect themselves from fecal disease, malaria, and tuberculosis. School plays and stories featuring Jamaican people speaking patois rather than formal English, and adult education campaigns that reached people with brochures and booklets featuring illustrations of Jamaicans and advice keyed to the island's setting communicated ideas about disease control. Benjamin Washburn, the Rockefeller agent in Jamaica, also built a public health establishment staffed by Afro-Jamaicans rather than by British officials.

Jamaicans learned that mosquitoes transmitted malaria and what to do to control mosquitoes in their own households and environs. They learned how to recognize that a member of the household had tuberculosis and what steps to take to protect themselves. Thus the country's survival gains in the 1920s and 1930s rested chiefly on things people learned to do for themselves. The advice they received came from the outside world, but the essential actions taken to reduce mortality from malaria, tuberculosis, and fecal disease came from Jamaicans.

Cubans benefited from economic development in the latter part of the nineteenth century and the first quarter of the twentieth, which enabled the government to spend more on health and education. Jamaica, by contrast, remained considerably poorer than Cuba in those decades. Its heyday as a plantation economy had been the eighteenth century. But in Jamaica, too, higher government spending on health and education compensated to some degree for what people could not themselves afford.

Jamaica's post–World War II economic boom, which rested initially on exploiting bauxite deposits and in the longer run mostly on tourism, elevated Jamaica between 1945 and 1972 to the status of a comparatively well-off poor country. Antibiotics and the new vaccines arrived in those years; hospitals were expanded; the primary school system grew nearly apace with the population; and secondary schools and a university were added. The hygiene curriculum was at first limited in reach to girls taking domestic arts courses and then removed. But by that point, in the 1940s, an entire generation had mastered their hygiene lessons: in the 1920s and 1930s school children learned lessons about disease avoidance and carried those lessons home to their parents; in the 1940s and 1950s those children, now parents, taught their own children these lessons, and they may also have negotiated more effectively for health services for their children. Indeed, throughout this early period most Jamaican households were headed by women who made their own decisions about what to do when a child was sick, within the limits of their resources. Malaria, tuberculosis, and fecal disease did not reemerge, and the diseases that could be treated with antibiotics, especially tuberculosis and typhoid fever, had already, before the arrival of the new medications, declined to a small fraction of their earlier importance as causes of death.

Dissatisfied with the hospital-based health care system inherited from British rule, after independence in 1962 Jamaicans expanded the number and accessibility of primary care facilities. A system of some forty district medical officers had been created in 1867; in the 1960s and 1970s Jamaica built hundreds of clinics and staffed them with health workers who received rudimentary training meant to enable them to perform basic care and triage, sending serious cases on to secondary and tertiary care institutions, and to advise pregnant women about childbirth and mothers about infant and child care. Jamaicans no longer had to travel more than a few miles, at most, to find health care of this quality. Ironically, this primary health care system was directed at the maladies of childhood and youth at a moment when Jamaica's disease profile had already begun shifting toward the degenerative organ diseases of older adulthood.

Jamaica's economic downturn in the years 1973–87 and the failure thereafter to revive economic growth led many observers to predict that infant mortality would increase and that some familiar communicable diseases would return. Globalization, which threatened to overwhelm Jamaican manufacturers, and insistence from the World Bank and the International Monetary Fund that the country reduce its debt, its deficit, and the size of its public sector likewise elevated anxieties about the country's good health status. Could Jamaica remain a poor country where people nevertheless lived long lives if public spending had to be curtailed? But survival continued to improve, after discounting the overly optimistic estimates made by government agencies. By 2002 life expectancy was probably not as high as the World Bank estimate of 75.7 years, but Jamaica remained an exceptional case of a low-income country with extraordinary survival.

Conclusion

In disease suppression, both Cuba and Jamaica made important progress in reducing malaria morbidity and mortality by controlling malarial mosquitoes decades before the introduction of DDT. That their successes were sustained rather than temporary may be owing in part to the circumstance of their being small island nations, thus without the problem of neighbors whose mosquito populations remained uncontrolled. The essential step toward mosquito control in both countries began with the organization of campaigns involving clearance and filling of sites where mosquitoes may lurk and breed around houses; some drainage programs, although large-scale drainage was beyond the financial reach of either; and the use of larvicides and insecticides plus larvae-eating fish. Parts of this program were designed by U.S. Army health authorities in Cuba in 1899 and 1900 against *Aedes aegypti* and yellow fever, and then enlarged to include steps appropriate to the breeding and feeding sites of the malaria-carrying anopheles and its preferred habitats. Benjamin Washburn, the Rockefeller Foundation agent in Jamaica, incorporated similar steps into the anti-anopheles program he urged upon Jamaicans, in cooperation with British authorities.

In Cuba, U.S. health authorities set out to improve water safety and human waste disposal in Havana, but did little for the rest of the island. Mortality from fecal disease declined sharply in Havana in the early years of this program, but for other areas diarrheal diseases remained an important cause of death for some decades thereafter. In Jamaica, in contrast, improvements to Kingston's water and sewage disposal system were matched by an aggressive and successful campaign to persuade rural Jamaicans, who made up most of the populace, to build latrines, maintain them and keep them clean, and use them. One of the arguments that Washburn and his Jamaican teams used was the threat of hookworm. Films and lurid verbal descriptions of how the small parasite enters the skin (usually between the toes) and multiplies to produce enervation and anemia, preserved specimens, and widespread experience with infection persuaded Jamaicans that they should give up their habit of defecating in the bush and use latrines.

In the case of tuberculosis, U.S. authorities had an isolation hospital built in Cuba and many Cubans with active cases of tuberculosis were removed from their homes and workplaces. Isolation in the hospital reduced exposure to the disease among family members, neighbors, and workmates. Jamaicans had the same idea, but until 1940 managed only to isolate a few of the sick in tuberculosis wards of district hospitals and a small unit in Kingston. In Jamaica the campaign against tuberculosis relied more heavily on informing people about how to recognize the disease, through house-to-house visits by public health nurses and adult health education; persuading people to house the sick separately, such as in huts attached to their dwellings; and asking people to cough, spit, and sneeze into handkerchiefs that were disinfected or burned after use. That was apparently enough, for tuberculosis mortality fell most rapidly in the 1930s.

Outside health authorities, in Cuba from the United States and in Jamaica from Britain and the United States, introduced ideas about germ theory, the role of vectors in transmitting some diseases, public health means of disease control, and steps people could take to protect themselves against disease. Cuban doctors accepted U.S. innovations with considerable grace and enthusiasm, which good progress at disease control seemed to justify. In Jamaica there was some cooperation from British health authorities, but there the main successes depended on the cooperation of the people and the creation of a public health establishment staffed by Jamaicans rather than by the British or by Americans.

In both countries the foundations laid early on, in Cuba in the period 1900–1925 and in Jamaica from the 1910s to the 1940s, initiated gains in survival and supported gains in the longer run. After 1959 Castro managed to maintain gains in life expectancy, and to democratize the educational and health systems. Jamaica managed to sustain its gains even through the long period of economic malaise that has persisted since the mid-1970s.

Political and economic systems seem to have had remarkably little impact on the life expectancy history of either Cuba or Jamaica. In Cuba a U.S.-dominated colonial system launched gains, which persisted even during the era of corrupt dictatorship and crony capitalism in the 1940s and 1950s. Castro revived the intention to improve the public's health, especially that of Afro-Cubans, under a benevolent communist dictatorship. In Jamaica the British colonialists laid the foundations of education and medical care but restricted Jamaican capitalism to an inferior, dependent position. There intervention by the Rockefeller Foundation and a public health alliance between the Americans and Jamaicans reduced risks from the leading causes of death. Survival gains continued after self-government was attained in 1944, through independence in 1962, and even during the ineffectual regimes, rising violence, and corruption of the 1970s and afterwards. In both countries life expectancy continued to improve in the 1990s and into the new century, despite economic turmoil and weak political leadership, even though observers in both countries worried that the underlying resources that permitted this continuing improvement would soon be exhausted.

Public health improvements played the leading role in both Cuba and Jamaica in the early period of survival progress, up to the 1950s, led in Cuba by the control of mosquitoes, smallpox vaccinations, and the isolation of people with tuberculosis, and in Jamaica by mosquito control, latrine-building, and education of people about how to recognize tuberculosis and protect themselves from a family member or close associate with the disease. In Jamaica schooling also played a part, building on the expansion of primary education that began in the 1890s and rising proportions of girls in school, though the effects of rising educational attainment were not felt until the 1920s. There self-reliance mattered more than contributions from the outside, either Britain or the United States, toward building public health institutions.

In both Cuba and Jamaica the 1960s and 1970s saw greater emphasis on medicine and egalitarian access to health care facilities. Jamaica invested comparatively meager amounts in building a system, the base of which consisted of numerous community health aides with a few years training, whereas Cuba trained many new physicians, taught the physicians how to communicate with people with little or no of schooling, and made an explicit point of reducing inequalities in health care based on race, region of residence, and income. Both countries also built medical education facilities and trained these higher numbers of health providers on their own.

CHAPTER 7

The Soviet and Chinese Models of Social Development

A large number of countries followed the communist-based social development model of the Soviet Union, either voluntarily or involuntarily, as members of the Soviet bloc, and additional countries followed the Chinese variation on the Soviet model.[1] All the countries that pursued these models for several decades managed to elevate life expectancy much faster and to a much higher level than could be predicted from the level of GDPpc or other measures of economic activity.[2] These countries practiced a form of authoritarian socialism, in which strong central political authority was brought to bear, and the central authority made choices largely on its own about which policies to adopt and how to implement them.

Typically the Soviet Union and the other communist countries made especially rapid gains in life expectancy between 1945 and 1960 or, in the case of China, between the late 1940s and the late 1960s. Thus there was a particular period of exceptional progress, and it is worth focusing both on prior steps that prepared the way for this rapid progress and on the policies pursued in the years of rapid improvement.

While the chapter focuses on the Soviet Union and China, it also touches on the interesting case of Albania and includes some information on Ukraine, whose history of longevity in some ways differs from and in others reflects that of Russia.[3] Figure 24 surveys the life expectancy record in these countries. All initiated health transitions before the 1940s, but made meager progress, often interrupted by chaotic events that caused mortality to surge temporarily.

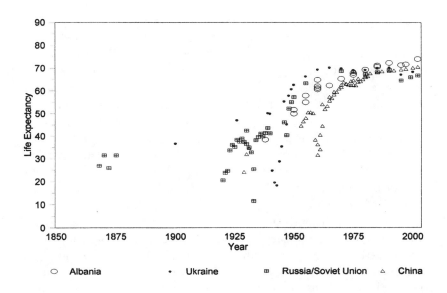

FIGURE 24. Life expectancy estimates for four communist countries, 1868–2000. For Russia/Soviet Union, Albania, and Ukraine, estimates are reported only for every fifth year 1950–95; more detail may be found in the sources. The detail has been kept for China in this period because there was greater year-to-year variation. SOURCES: *For Russia / Soviet Union:* Serguei Adamets, "Famine in Nineteenth-and Twentieth-Century Russia: Mortality by Age, Cause, and Gender," in *Famine Demography: Perspectives from the Past and Present,* ed. Tim Dyson and Cormac Ó Gráda (Oxford: Oxford University Press, 2002), pp. 158–80; Eugenii Andreev, Leonid Darskij, and Tatiana Kharkova, "L'histoire de la population de l'URSS 1920–1959," *Annales de démographie historique* (1992): 61–150; Vladimir M. Shkolnikov, and France Meslé, "The Russian Epidemiological Crisis as Mirrored by Mortality Trends," in *Russia's Demographic 'Crisis,'* ed. Julie DaVanzo and Gwendolyn Farnsworth (Santa Monica, CA: RAND, 1996), pp. 113–62; Vladimir Shkolnikov, France Meslé, and Jacques Vallin, "La crise sanitaire en Russie. I. Tendances récentes de l'espérance de vie et des causes de décès de 1970 à 1993," *Population* 50 (1995): 907–42; and Shkolnikov, Meslé, and Vallin, "La crise sanitaire en Russie. II. Évolution des causes de décès: comparaison avec la France et l'Angleterre (1970–1993)," *Population* 50 (1995): 945–82. *For Albania:* Arjan Gjonça, *Communism, Health and Lifestyle: The Paradox of Mortality Transition in Albania, 1950–1990* (Westport, CT: Greenwood Press, 2001), pp. 181–82; Ermelinda Meksi and Gianpiero Dalla Zuanna, "La mortalité générale en Albanie (1950–1990)," *Population* 49 (1994): 607–35; United Nations, *Demographic Yearbook: Historical Supplement 1948–1997* CD-ROM (New York: Department of Economic and Social Affairs, Statistical Office, United Nations, n.d.); and World Bank, *World Development Indicators 2004 on CD-ROM* (Washington: World Bank, 2004). *For Ukraine:* France Meslé and Jacques Vallin, *Mortalité et causes de décès en Ukraine au XXe siècle* (Paris: Institut national d'études démographiques, 2003). *For China:* Judith Banister and Kenneth Hill, "Mortality in China 1964–2000," *Population Studies* 58 (2004): 55–75; John Caldwell et al., "Population Trends in China—A Perspective Provided by the 1982 Census," in *A Census of One Billion People,* ed. Chengrui Li (Hong Kong: Economic Information and Agency, 1986), pp. 352–91; Sheng Luo, "Reconstruction of Life Tables and Age Distributions for the Population of China, by Year, from 1953 to 1982" (PhD diss., University of Pennsylvania, 1988); and World Bank, *World Development Indicators 2004 on CD-ROM* (Washington: World Bank, 2004).

European Russia appears to have begun its health transition in the years 1890–1910, but the transition was interrupted by World War I, and then, for the new Soviet Union, by the 1918–19 influenza epidemic, the civil war that ended in 1920, the combination of typhus and typhoid fever epidemics and famine in 1920–22, the agricultural crisis surrounding 1929 collectivization, the 1932–34 and 1946–47 famines, Stalin's purges of 1937–41, and World War II in 1941–45. During the 1920s infant mortality dropped from about 250 per 1,000 live births to about 180, but did not decline much further until the period from the late 1940s to 1960, when it dropped from about 175 to between 35 and 40.[4] Rural infant mortality remained lower than urban until after 1970, according to Natalia Kseno-fontova's corrected estimates.[5] But Soviet economic development was ac-companied by urbanization, with the fraction of the population living in urban areas rising from 15 percent in 1897 to 39 percent in 1950 and 49 percent in 1960. Thus, because, at least for infants, survival prospects were better in the countryside, urbanization tended for a long time to reduce life expectancy.

If rapid progress came later, there is nevertheless much that is note-worthy about the years 1910 to 1945. Available estimates of life expectancy suggest that recoveries from each crisis that Russia and the Soviet Union faced were not just rapid but also that each time they tended to carry sur-vival to a slightly higher level that was then sustained. As a part of the So-viet Union particularly exposed to these crises, Ukraine followed a simi-lar path and is of particular interest because estimates of survival during World War II are available only for Ukraine; those suggest that life ex-pectancy dropped as low as 18.2 years in 1943.[6]

The earliest estimate for Albania, for 1938, puts life expectancy some-where below 38.3 years, "below" because the deaths on which this estimate is based are known to have been underreported. Arjan Gjonça argues that survival gains began before 1930. In the 1930s Albania was a mostly agrar-ian society, where malaria and tuberculosis caused many deaths. Some development of mining and manufacturing had begun, but there is very little in the descriptive evidence to suggest any basis for survival gains.[7] Nevertheless, the high life expectancy level achieved by 1950, 50 to 52 years, certainly implies an earlier beginning period, presumably before World War II and before the disruptive Italo-German occupation of 1939–44. The communist regime that took power in 1944 set out to transform the country by adopting a Stalinist program, the main elements of which per-sisted through Albania's period of isolation from 1978 to 1990. Aid from the Soviet Union and East European countries and malaria eradication using DDT allowed Albania to make especially rapid gains in survival in the late 1940s and 1950s. With the shift from Soviet to Chinese sponsorship in 1961–62 and the turn toward isolation in 1978, however, life expectancy stagnated.[8]

After a period of rapid economic growth in Albania, from 1990 to 1996, a financial collapse occurred. Many social facilities were destroyed during a period of near anarchy.[9] Government spending on health and education was already contracting in 1992–95, making it difficult to reconcile descriptive information about Albanian society or the economy with the government's claims of continuing gains in life expectancy.

A number of estimates have been ventured for China's life expectancy around 1930, with the spread ranging from 24.2 to 34.7 years.[10] At the time, according to one report, about 25 percent of all deaths were due to fecal disease and a further 10 to 15 percent to tuberculosis; malaria was also a significant cause of death, but limited to certain regions.[11] If the higher estimates of life expectancy are accurate, then it appears that China initiated gains in the 1920s, during a period of economic expansion and, by the mid-1930s, significant investments in public health and education.[12] The Japanese war and the Chinese civil war soon interrupted, so that from 1937 to 1949 survival rates were much poorer. Mao's seizure of power in 1949 inaugurated a period in which the national will was turned toward a Maoist model of social development, and life expectancy gains were particularly rapid until 1959.[13]

In the Soviet Union and its successor states, the rapid gains up to about 1960 were followed by a long period of fluctuation around the level of life expectancy already attained, 68 to 70 years.[14] China's gains were briefly negated with the famine of 1959–61 that followed the Great Leap Forward, then rebounded during the 1970s; China reached the 68 to 70 level in the late 1980s and thereafter found further gains difficult to make. Among these countries, only Albania broke with this pattern. There in the late 1990s life expectancy rose once more, reaching 73.7 to 74 years in 2002. A healthier lifestyle and perhaps also the continuing poverty of the country, which limited tobacco and alcohol use and thus their disease sequelae, and few deaths from motor vehicle accidents, allowed Albania to take the life expectancy lead among these countries toward the end of the 1990s.

Figure 25 reports Maddison's estimates of GDPpc for these countries. Economic growth was pronounced in the 1950s and 1960s, which made resources available for new policy initiatives. In all four cases consumer choices were less important in how these resources were allocated than were decisions made by the central authorities.

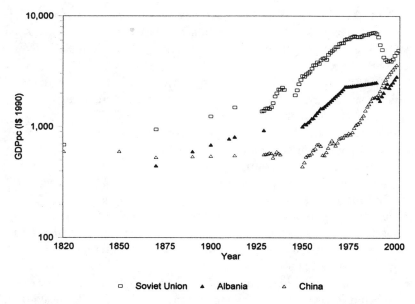

FIGURE 25. Gross domestic product per capita (GDPpc) in 1900 international dollars (I$) in three communist countries, 1820–2000. GDPpc appears in a logarithmic scale in order to compress information and to show the pace of change.
SOURCE: Angus Maddison, *The World Economy: Historical Statistics* (Paris: Development Center of the Organization for Economic Cooperation and Development, 2003), pp. 100–101, 180–84.

Soviet bloc countries in general followed a similar pattern in life expectancy gains. During the rapid improvements of 1945–60 Bulgaria, Czechoslovakia, Hungary, Poland, and Romania reached a plateau of 67 to 70 years that they maintained thereafter up to and through the 1989–91 breakup of the Soviet bloc. Thus the Soviet model, and the variations on it followed by Albania and China, seem to have served well in controlling communicable diseases and reducing infant mortality, but to have been less effective at managing chronic organ diseases, alcoholism, and deaths from injuries.[15] In addition, since 1989 authorities report the reappearance in the Russian Federation of some communicable diseases, including diphtheria.

When the American physician William A. Knaus reflected on his 1973–74 visit to the Soviet Union, he drew a contrast between individual freedom in the United States and state decision-making on behalf of the individual in the Soviet Union. "In the United States . . . responsibility for and decisions about personal health . . . rest with the individual," who ". . . is held to account for personal habits relating to his or her health and for seeking medical care when and if it is needed," while "in the Soviet Union, 'the health of each citizen is regarded not only as his personal affair but as part of the national wealth.'"[16] Every medical system places most responsibility for initiating contact with health providers on the individual, who decides when he or she is sick, or sick enough, to see a doctor. No-cost care in the Soviet Union made that an easier decision to take, Knaus observed. But it is also true that a contrast should be drawn between the reluctance of the public sector in the United States and many other noncommunist countries to invest in community health or to intrude on the individual's health practices and the intrusiveness of the Soviet system. The communist countries shed this reluctance, not because they invested more heavily in public health, for they did not initially, but because they did not need to respect individual freedom. As a result, they could much more forcefully instruct people to practice community health. Whereas capitalist countries sometimes counted on the enthusiasm of the populace to change the public's health behavior, as both Jamaica and Mexico did in the 1920s and 1930s, communist countries could oblige compliance even in the face of limited choices and surly resistance.

The Soviet Model

In the years immediately after the 1917 revolution, and especially from 1928, when the first five-year plan was implemented, the Soviet Union reorganized the economy, adopting central planning; public ownership of manufacturing, transport, and many other activities; and controlled markets. Along a parallel track and inspired by Lenin's 1920 speech to the Young Communist League, the revolutionaries altered social goals and policies. To replace the social status quo, with its sharply defined hierarchy of wealth, political authority, education, and social power, the new regime set out to destroy the old elites and to engage a much wider swath of the populace in the ongoing revolution aimed at making the new Soviet citizen. Central planning incorporated specific objectives in literacy and education, medicine, child health, and public health and, through moral or ideological education, the explicit aim of changing behavior.

From the perspective of disease, the task was substantial. Official statistics reporting cases of infectious diseases for the period 1913–46 show a profile including smallpox, cholera, typhoid fever, malaria (the most commonplace of all reported disease in the early 1930s),[17] tuberculosis, whooping cough, scarlet fever, typhus, and others. Among those only smallpox and cholera were eradicated, or nearly eradicated, during that period. Malaria control initially deteriorated because the Soviet Union imported less quinine and used inferior substitutes to manage the fever and debility associated with this disease.[18]

In 1919 the Soviet Union embarked on simultaneous campaigns aimed at social and economic development, with education and literacy being a centerpiece of social development. The zemstvos, or local assemblies, of the tsarist regime, introduced as part of a reform in the 1860s, had promoted rural education and had made some progress in elevating levels of literacy. By 1914 more than half of school-age children were enrolled in primary schools.[19] Between the censuses of 1897 and 1926 (there were none in the interim) literacy at ages 9–49 rose from 28.4 to 56.6 percent. By 1939 the rate reached 87 percent, and by 1959, 96 percent. In the meantime female literacy advanced much faster than male, rising from 17 percent of this age group in 1897 to 43 percent in 1926, 82 percent in 1939, and 98 percent in 1959, when it exceeded the level of male literacy.[20]

It proved much easier to make bold plans—and to publish exaggerated statistics—than actually to transform education, however, especially in circumstances in which, as in the 1920s, teachers at all levels were suspect because of their pre-revolutionary class position. The Bolsheviks aimed to provide education for the masses, meaning not just the few years of schooling required to teach people how to read and write, but advanced technical education from which the children of industrial workers and peasants would rise to take places in the new regime as engineers, doctors, and teachers. Schools were expected "to prepare the new Soviet person capable of completing the transition to communism,"[21] a goal taken as seriously by many people into the 1970s as in the 1920s. Up to the late 1920s the campaign for education and literacy was pushed mostly in the cities. Then, simultaneously with collectivization, began the rural part of the campaign. A 1930 law made three years of education compulsory, but the rural program was underfunded. Peasants remained hostile toward and suspicious of many teachers. A 1931 curriculum reform moved away from innovations made earlier, which included hygiene education, and back to a traditional curriculum. Elementary and secondary enrollments rose rapidly between 1928 and 1932 and continued to rise thereafter, while the Soviets trained an entire generation of new teachers, often drafting graduates of secondary schools who had not had any pedagogic training.[22] The 1939 census indicates that much had been accomplished in making peasants literate, but the plans and promises for a worker and peasant intelligentsia had not yet been realized.[23]

These weaknesses notwithstanding, the Soviet model in education called for universal literacy, at least for the younger generation, a massive expansion of technical and higher education, adult education, and the schooling of females as readily as males. Although educational progress was interrupted by World War II, it resumed in the late 1940s. The Soviet Union reached the goal of mass literacy faster than any other country had, up to the 1950s, and that success constituted part of its appeal to newly independent countries of the late 1940s and 1960s considering how to set and reach their own objectives.[24]

Before the 1917 revolution, health services had been oriented toward cities, although the zemstvos sought with some success to build rural health facilities.[25] During the 1920s most improvements in the health system still favored city dwellers, but investment in rural medicine increased in the 1930s, as more hospitals were built and more medical practitioners added. No more than slow progress was made in adding higher-level services until the period 1947–60, when the ratio of doctors per 10,000 people rose from under 14 to 19, and of hospital beds per 10,000 from under 56 to 80.[26] Knaus remarked: "Most of the new Soviet hospitals [of the 1930s] were simply large rooms filled with beds," and equipment and medications were in short supply.[27] In the meantime the Soviet Union trained large numbers of auxiliary medical practitioners—including midwives, pediatric nurses, and public health nurses—to supplement or replace the feldshers (informally trained practitioners) of the pre-revolutionary period, and expanded the number of medical stations offering basic treatment, vaccinations, and infant and maternal care.[28] Throughout this prewar period Soviet medicine emphasized larger numbers of medical personnel rather than first-class medical facilities; by 1940 or 1941 there were more than 34,500 health centers and 95,000 feldshers. The Soviet medical school curriculum placed greater weight on public health and disease prevention than did its Western counterpart.

In health, as in education, more was planned or proposed than achieved. In 1918 the Soviets made smallpox vaccination compulsory, announced one campaign against tuberculosis and another to promote the welfare of mothers and children, and proposed hygiene instruction for the general population. Into the 1930s, however, urban areas and industrial workers benefited from medical advances much more than did rural areas and peasants.[29] Samuel C. Ramer reports than in 1930 nearly 90 percent of "peasant women still gave birth either alone or with the help of a traditional midwife."[30]

In medicine the Soviet model consisted, in theory, of democratic and free access to health care for the entire population, albeit to care often lacking technological equipment, up-to-date medicines, and physicians trained to a West European standard (which would not be achieved until the 1950s).[31] Reliance on the thousands of auxiliary medical providers trained in the Soviet model was an important factor in the Soviet Union's promotion of primary health care at WHO meetings and, ultimately, at Alma Ata in 1978, where delegates approved the goal of making rudimentary health care available to everyone across the globe.

Lenin dreamed of nurseries and kindergartens to tend and cultivate children in the new regime, in which women would join the ranks of workers, and of child health facilities that would help produce a new generation of Soviet people. A national system of child health facilities took decades to build. In the meantime the new regime did successfully promote health education for expectant mothers, home visits, advice bureaus, and milk kitchens, even as it also succeeded in getting mothers into the workplace.[32]

In public health the plans announced in 1918 anticipated a rapid adoption of the latest West European approaches. But resources in finance and personnel were simply inadequate. In 1922 the Soviets transferred funding of public health initiatives to local authorities, which led to a reduction of existing physician and hospital services rather than an expansion into sanitation, laboratory medicine, and other cutting edge areas of pubic health. The five-year plan initiated in 1928 conceived of a major expansion in public health activity as well as in medicine. But in 1930 only 23 of 508 cities in the Russian part of the Soviet Union had sewage systems, and most of the other plans also remained unfulfilled.[33]

A pension program was introduced 1927 and expanded in 1937 to include most workers, although not people working on farm collectives. Because of price instability thereafter, however, the pension paid was often too little to cover basic needs. Rising female labor force participation, which led to women contributing more directly to household earnings, and more years of schooling may have given women and mothers greater power in negotiating how household resources were spent.[34] Fertility declined some in the 1940s and persistently after 1950, which presumably added to the household resources that could be devoted to a smaller number of children in the Soviet Union. But Albania managed much the same pace of gains in survival amidst sharply rising female labor force participation and no decline in fertility.

In the Soviet Union the Soviet model remained more a set of aspirations than reality until the 1930s, when much more rapid progress was made in the health system and in improving survival than had been done in the 1920s. These plans were pursued once again after World War II, and it was then that their effects seem to have been felt most dramatically in improving population health and survival. Especially given the many crises of the 1920s and 1930s, achievements toward realizing this model by the mid-1950s must be counted as stunning, even heroic. The central element of the model lies in its attempt at social rather than material development, at improving education, health care, and child care rather than elevating the standard of living as defined in the West. In the Soviet Union this model was labor-intensive. Physical capital was meant to accumulate in mining and industry more than in schools, hospitals, and the other physical structures of social development. Its place was taken by human capital, including that of women.[35]

Albania at first copied the Soviet initiatives, adapting some to local needs.[36] There health aides filled a broader function than in the Soviet model, working in education as well as health and disease prevention, while DDT use in low-lying regions, plus some drainage and tillage improvements, eradicated malaria in the postwar period. Illiteracy, estimated at 80 percent in 1945, declined under the educational reform of 1946, which made four years of schooling compulsory and led to sharply rising school enrollments.

China

While the Soviet model was applied in Eastern Europe and Albania, and to some degree also in Vietnam, it influenced but did not comprise the central element of the social development policies that China adopted in 1949. Under its own version of communism, according to the best available estimates and to scholarly consensus, Maoist China made rapid progress in adding to survival almost immediately. Mortality dropped sharply across the 1950s, up to the famine of 1959–61 and again after that crisis. Many programs and policy initiatives have been linked to these sudden and impressive gains. But in the Western framework, in which institutional inputs bulk large, no single Chinese program, nor even the entire group of them, seems substantial enough to account for the scale of gains. One possibility is that life expectancy in China has been overstated at every point, beginning in the early 1950s.[37] Another possibility, which can be called the crisis-recovery thesis, is that rapid gains in the early 1950s were possible because Maoist China was to some degree restoring survival conditions that existed in the mid-1930s rather than breaking entirely new ground.

All authorities agree that the Chinese faced an unusually broad spectrum of diseases, including both tropical and temperate zone maladies. Judith Banister argues that mortality remained high, at around 40 deaths per 1,000, across the early decades of the twentieth century.[38] But her interpretation requires even more rapid gains in the 1950s for China to have reached the life expectancy level reported for the 1960s. According to the crisis-recovery thesis China, like the Soviet Union after each of its mortality crises, brought survival back up to the pre-crisis level and beyond by restoring earlier conditions after the difficult years 1937–49 while also introducing new initiatives. Ka-che Yip reports that the Chinese Communists took over and expanded on an earlier Nationalist health program begun in the 1920s.[39] That argument both supports the crisis-recovery interpretation and gives Chinese gains a cast influenced not just by Mao's interpretation of Soviet ideas but also by Western influences, including missionaries and the Rockefeller and Milbank Memorial Foundations, which attempted to develop medicine and public health in China between the late nineteenth century and the 1930s.[40]

The health programs and policies China adopted in 1949 and afterwards differ enough from those pursued by the Soviet Union to justify the idea of a Chinese model in health. Mao Zedong and his associates closely followed the Soviet model in economic development, in building socialism, and in entrusting leadership to a single person. But their own nationalism and an accurate sense that Chinese realities differed led them to adopt some distinctive approaches.[41] Specifically, while the national government set health policies from 1949, those policies were carried out at the county level and with county resources.[42]

In health, communist rule opened with a crash program of smallpox vaccination in 1949–52.[43] Up to the late 1950s the mass mobilization for environmental sanitation, launched in 1952 as the Patriotic Hygiene Campaign, comprised the central part of disease control programs. Since China lacked financial resources during and after the Korean War, to a degree that matched or exceeded the scarcity of such resources in the Soviet Union in the early 1920s, initiatives depended on human effort. These initiatives took three directions. First, the Patriotic Hygiene Campaign sought to cleanse the environment by cleaning up towns and cities, managing refuse and waste in urban and rural areas, and reducing breeding and feeding opportunities for disease vectors, especially rats, snails, lice, houseflies, and mosquitoes. State authorities pushed latrine building, alerted people to the role of human feces in disease propagation, encouraged composting of night soil before its use as fertilizer, and in general followed a household approach to sanitation.[44] Adults and children caught and trapped vast numbers of vermin and insects and killed them. Householders built latrines earlier than cities introduced waterborne sewage removal and treatment. Hygiene, sanitation, and health educa- tion programs had been organized in communist controlled areas in the 1940s, and the Patriotic Hygiene Campaign extended those to the entire country.[45] These programs mix Chinese inspiration with Western ideas familiar for their application in a number of low-income countries in the 1920s and 1930s.

Second, the campaign asked people to learn how to protect themselves against disease, using "continuous social pressure to induce changes in individual behavior and attitudes toward personal hygiene, environ- mental sanitation, and nutrition." Both of these approaches required ma- jor changes in day-to-day behavior and the assumption by the populace of responsibility for safeguarding their own health in what Peter Heller calls a strategy of self-reliance, but which might also be styled a strategy of regimentation and indoctrination. People were instructed about when they needed to boil water to destroy pathogens; from 1955 into the 1970s villagers were mobilized twice a year to dig new ditches or drain old ones and bury the top layer of dirt containing snails that potentially bore schis- tosomiasis; a few villagers were trained to identify certain diseases, in- cluding hookworm, and to select people needing treatment.[46] Thus the program of medical auxiliaries best known under the rubric "barefoot doc- tors" was preceded in the 1950s by brief training for large numbers of med- ical aides who staffed rural health units, provided maternal and child health services, and directed local hygiene and sanitation programs. China also revived the county-level hospital building program of the 1930s and built thousands of health clinics and health stations as well.[47]

Third, the Chinese, copying the Soviets, began a massive program to train physicians and medical aids and to build hospitals and clinics. Even though urban industrial workers were favored recipients of health care in China as they had been in the Soviet Union, the general population gained access to care from providers with formal, although sometimes quite brief, training, as well as to county-level hospitals. Chinese authorities also or- ganized mass vaccination campaigns to prevent smallpox, the forms of tuberculosis preventable by BCG vaccine, which was produced in China, diphtheria, and some other diseases. And China began to produce its own sulfa drugs, penicillin, the malaria drug Proguanil (an herbal remedy also known as Paludrine), and additional vaccines.

In the mid-1960s China shifted the orientation of its health campaign

toward providing services at the village level, expanding the smaller number of community health workers operating in the late 1950s into a vast
corps of briefly trained practitioners, the famous barefoot doctors. As early
as 1931 health workers had been given a one-year course to prepare them
to serve in the Red Army. A few years later, after the Long March, Mao
provided for training of civilian health workers as well in the three
provinces of north China under his control. Both those steps resemble
the transformation of pre-revolutionary feldshers into the community
health aides of the revolutionary period in Russia. But they also resemble the corps of health workers in Ding Xian and its region in the early
1930s, an area about a hundred miles south of Beijing that was under Nationalist control.[48] Thus the inspiration for China's use of briefly trained
medical auxiliaries remains uncertain.

Barefoot doctors, sometimes also called peasant doctors, treated people
for minor ailments, decided who should be sent to the commune hospital, gave immunizations, and dispensed medicines, at first mostly traditional herbal remedies, but after 1970 Western drugs manufactured in
China as well.[49] They also advised people about how to avoid disease, led
local health education campaigns, and took over direction of public
health efforts under the Patriotic Hygiene Campaign. In an exceptionally intrusive process of persistent intervention, women barefoot doctors
coached women through pregnancies, assisted at childbirth, and taught
new mothers how to care for their infants. Worker doctors with similarly
brief training filled a like role in urban factories; and Red Guard doctors,
mostly women trained for ten days, worked for a few years from the mid-
1960s at the street level, organizing people for hygiene campaigns, making sure children got their immunizations, overseeing family planning,
and assisting health station doctors.[50] More midwives were trained and
they attended more births and gave mothers advice about how to care for
infants. China did not, before the late 1970s, have much in the way of a
supply of antibiotics.[51] Thus, although the term *barefoot doctor* suggests
an emphasis on health care, there was rather little that these medical aids
could do to treat sickness. Rather, Chinese efforts in the era of the barefoot doctors were directed more toward disease prevention—public
health and advising individuals what they might do to prevent or manage disease—than toward treatment and cure.[52]

In the meantime China expanded its health facilities and trained many
physicians, including the barefoot doctors, in a mixture of traditional and
Western medicine.[53] By the 1970s urban areas had health facilities re-
sembling those in the Soviet Union while rural areas relied on barefoot
doctors, county hospitals, and the Cooperative Medical System.[54]

In schooling in the early 1950s China had to contend with a dearth of teachers, especially of teachers sympathetic to the new regime, which meant that primary schools were mostly staffed by people who had too few years of education to qualify for certification. Mao's regime adopted five policies for the educational system: ideological training, economic reorientation, attitudes sympathetic to Soviet Russia, attitudes unsympathetic to the United States, and improvement of health. In the school and in adult education programs these objectives competed to some degree with training in literacy and numeracy. But in any case many adults sought to learn to read, and many more children attended school than had done so before 1949.[55]

After some initial gains, literacy deteriorated from about 1956, even before the beginning of the Cultural Revolution during which many schools were closed. Vilma Seeberg estimates literacy among people aged 16 and up at 34.2 percent in 1952, declining to 10.6 percent in the early 1970s, with much of this sharp decline resulting from the disruption of education during Japanese occupation and the civil war. (These events would not be felt in literacy statistics for people aged 16 and up until children born in the late 1930s and 1940s reached age 16).[56] The World Bank, using official estimates, puts literacy at 53 percent in 1970, rising to 91 percent in 2000.[57] The disagreement is about what happened between 1956 and 1970, and too little reliable information is available to resolve it.[58] Literacy in 1970 may actually have been little or no higher than it was in 1949, around 32 percent of people over 12. Or it may be that a higher proportion of people could read and write a few hundred characters, but not the minimum number of four to six thousand counted as literacy. In any case, it is difficult, outside government propaganda, to find arguments that literacy gains coincided with gains in survival before the 1970s. By the 1990s, however, most children at ages 6–16 were enrolled in school.

The effectiveness of the Chinese approach toward improving survival relied in some measure on a Maoist reorganization of community life that featured neighborhood, village, and workplace units, the *danwei,* supervised by party cadres through whom members of the unit obtained health care as well as housing and other benefits. Organized in the 1950s, the danwei were used to make sure that individuals and the work unit acted in harmony with the aims of the communist party and, when they did, to provide social support. These work units would later, under the one-child campaign, be used successfully to monitor reproduction and guide people who wanted more than one child toward obedience.[59]

In its economic reforms of the 1980s and 1990s, China dismantled most features of the scheme that had allowed it to achieve one of the most rapid transitions from low to high life expectancy.[60] By the 1980s China had nearly completed its transition from conditions of around 1930, in which fecal disease, tuberculosis, malaria (in the south), and other communicable diseases dominated the cause-of-death profile and most deaths occurred in infancy or childhood, to the point where those diseases had waned sharply in importance, to be replaced by the chronic diseases of middle and old age.[61] But at that point, with life expectancy at 68, gains effectively ceased.

In particular, the new policy quickly shifted to an open market health system while moving much more gradually toward capitalism and open markets in other sectors of the economy. China abandoned subsidies for medical costs in rural areas and called for peasants to pay for health services. Barefoot doctors suddenly lost their jobs—and much of their influence—and had to try to support themselves by charging fees for services. Local public health and health education programs lost funding from the central government. At the same time, public funding for more specialized medicine, including hospitals, also decreased.[62] The danwei system, with its social controls, was disintegrating by the 1990s, although China still managed to prevent most rural dwellers from moving to cities. This probably played a role in income distribution becoming more skew, favoring urban over rural residents.[63]

Conclusion

The Chinese model for improving survival relied heavily on individual- and household-level improvements in hygiene and changes in behavior; on the mobilization of the population for public health initiatives in the Patriotic Hygiene Campaign; on universal access introduced in the 1960s to briefly trained barefoot doctors and their immunizations, advice on sanitation and health behavior, and selection of people needing skilled care; and on regimentation in the pursuit of objectives set by state authorities. These programs and policies achieved exceptionally rapid change in controlling disease risks. Mao's regime probably reduced population literacy but at the same time elevated how much ordinary people knew about how to protect themselves against disease risks. China's gains in survival in the 1950s and 1960s coincided with the introduction and elaboration of these programs and policies. And the deterioration of health in the 1980s, which took the form of higher mortality in rural than urban areas and of a national stagnation in life expectancy at 68 to 70 years and infant mortality at about 40 deaths per 1,000 live births, coincided with the dismantling of these programs and policies.[64]

In contrast, the Soviet model emphasized medical education that focused on public health, hospitals, general population literacy, a concentration of resources on maternal and child health, and egalitarian access to health care and education. Smallpox seems to have been controlled in the 1920s, but malaria remained a major cause of death and a major comorbidity into the 1940s. Urbanization long played a negative role in the Soviet Union, with higher infant mortality in cities in the period up to about 1960. Schooling also proceeded slowly, especially in the pace at which literacy and educational attainment among females caught up with that among males. But the Soviet regime was successful for a longer time, from the 1920s into the 1970s, at persuading many people to adapt to its socialist goals.

It is difficult to imagine in either case that the populace would have elected to invest human capital, time (in China), or public resources (in the Soviet Union) in these ways had such decisions been left up to them. Nevertheless, these state-enforced initiatives, which mixed some enthusiasm for socialism with a substantial measure of social pressure and authoritarian discipline, produced rapid improvement, especially in China.

Except in Albania, however, progress in survival faltered in the 1960s and 1970s. Neither the foundations laid in the Soviet Union and China in the 1920s and 1930s nor the improvements on those foundations made in the late 1940s and 1950s proved sufficient to sustain gains thereafter. Central authorities could mobilize the people to pursue health goals and for a time command acceptance of the goals they set, but their approach proved much less resistant to deterioration than what was achieved in Cuba and Jamaica, to cite just two other examples. Also, in the Soviet Union and even more so in China and Albania, official claims about education and literacy allege much faster progress than actually occurred. Thus, given the lag to be expected between rising schooling rates and a payoff in health, literacy and schooling themselves appear to have contributed little to improvements in survival until the 1950s in the Soviet Union and later still in Albania and China.

CHAPTER 8

Oil-Rich Lands

This chapter considers the experience of five countries in the Middle East (Iran, Iraq, Kuwait, Oman, and Saudi Arabia), two in North Africa (Algeria and Libya), and one in South America (Venezuela). In all eight, commercial production from oil reserves preceded or came in the early stages of gains in survival, occurred on a large scale, and produced resources that the public sector could use to advance community health.

The oil-rich countries are an exceptional case. They were all low-income countries when oil was first produced, but in a series of occasional and unpredictable spikes in income, oil sales raised them into the middle-income category. In times of atypically high petroleum prices, some of them even gained high-income status, though these periods lasted only as long as the high oil prices. Commercial exploitation of oil produced the initial spike. For some oil-rich countries new agreements on sharing oil revenues with the corporations or entities that actually extracted the petroleum gave the country a larger share of revenues and produced subsequent surges. For all of them the oil shock of 1975 produced another spike. (Of course, lower prices for oil on the world market might undermine plans made in the heady days of high prices.) And significantly, extracting government revenues from mineral reserves, rather than from taxes on the economic activity of their people, allowed the leaders of these generally autocratic countries to make decisions about how to allocate public spending with little reference to the wishes of subjects and citizens. In sum, each of the oil-rich countries had at least two opportunities to decide how to spend vast new sums, in the Middle East and North Africa without any com-

TABLE 11. Development of Oil Resources in 8 Countries

Country (year of independence, from)	Year Oil Discovered	Year Commercial Production of Oil Began	Proven Oil Reserves, January 2002 (billions of barrels)	Population, mid-2004 (millions)	Reserves per capita (barrels)
Algeria (1962, France)	1956	n.a.	13.1	32.1	408
Iran	1904	1908	94.4	69.0	1,368
Iraq (1932, League of Nations mandate under UK)	1927	about 1929	113.8	25.4	4,480
Kuwait (1961, United Kingdom)	1938	1946	97.7	2.3	42,478
Libya (1951, Italy)	1958	1961	29.8	5.6	5,321
Oman	1964	1967	5.7	2.9	1,966
Saudi Arabia	1932	1938	261.7	25.8	10,143
Venezuela (1811, Spain)	1860s	1918	64.0	25.0	2,560

SOURCES: *oil reserves:* United States, Central Intelligence Agency, *World Factbook 2003* at http://www.capitals.com/rankorder/2178rank.html; *population*: from United States, Central Intelligence Agency, *World Factbook 2004* at http://www.odci.gov/cia/publications/factbook/index.html.

pulsion to refer decisions to the public or, in Venezuela (and Mexico, where oil also played a role; see chapter 9), with only limited or episodic reference to the people's wishes. In other words, these countries had opportunities to make spending decisions denied most other lands, where it has usually been more difficult to divorce spending decisions from the will of taxpayers and the limits of less elastic revenues—or, as in communist nations, the demands of Marxist ideology and planning decisions. How, then, did population health fare from the decisions they made?

Table 11 lists the eight countries, dates the beginning of commercial production of oil, reports the scale of oil reserves in 2002, and gives the approximate per capita scale of those reserves. These eight all rank in the top twenty countries in proven oil reserves, as estimated by the U.S. Central Intelligence Agency for January 2002. At least from the 1960s, the most extensively documented case among these eight is Oman, which is also one of the most interesting cases because of its exceedingly rapid pace of survival gains.

Oman

Oman moved from a low- to a middle-income country between the early 1960s and the 1980s, according to World Bank estimates of GDPpc. UN and World Bank estimates of life expectancy both indicate that gains in survival began earlier, probably in the 1940s or 1950s.[1] But, as discussion below will show, life expectancy gains may actually have begun as late as the 1970s.

Western travelers, missionaries, and British officials working for the sultan of Oman characterized the country in the period 1930–60 as a land of deep poverty and widespread disease, lacking sanitary facilities, safe water, adequate housing, schools, or other amenities important to population health. Paul Harrison, an American physician who served for some years as a missionary doctor in a suburb of the capital, Muscat, in the 1920s and 1930s found dysentery, malaria, and trachoma to be the most common diseases in a population with "very poor health" owing chiefly to poverty, and high infant mortality owing chiefly to poor sanitation. Other authorities discuss tuberculosis, schistosomiasis (also called bilharzia), cholera, bubonic plague, and skin sores, plus protein and calorie malnutrition. Harrison explained the dense fly population not as a product of flies feeding and breeding at refuse sites, but of people depositing human feces here and there, creating a multitude of breeding and feeding sites. He recognized the theoretical utility of boiling water, but regarded that as an impractical thing to do, given meager supplies of water and fuel.[2]

Raymond O'Shea, who served at a Royal Air Force base built during World War II in an inland area called Trucial Oman (later part of the United Arab Emirates), repeated many of Harrison's points and added that the villages he saw lacked any arrangements for drainage or sanitation and were also without roads or schools. He also reported that slavery and the slave trade continued.[3] The three main cities, Muscat, Muttrah, and Salalah, certainly lacked most public health amenities as late as 1940, so that travelers did not distinguish between public health conditions in urban and rural areas. Nevertheless, villages, where most people lived, may have been healthier than the cities if only because settlement was so sparse.

Visitors also described some grounds for optimism, which allow the possibility that gains in life expectancy may have begun as early as the 1940s. Medical missionaries arrived in 1909, opening a women's dispensary in Muscat in 1913. Harrison, who founded his missionary hospital in 1935, noted that some people were beginning to use mosquito nets, that latrines built in the neighborhood of the mission hospital reduced waterborne-disease in that area, that some children were vaccinated against smallpox, and that secular schools were being set up, but he had more to say about the untapped potential to teach people about sanitation, child care, and other things important for health and survival. The British, who then regarded Oman as within of their sphere of influence, implemented some sanitary provisions at Muscat and set up quarantine facilities. A number of schools instructed students in the Quran. The first non-Quranic school seems to have been a missionary school opened in 1897; by the early 1960s Lebanese and Palestinian teachers instructed at a government elementary school in Muscat and two other primary schools, one at Muttrah and the other at Salalah. The Indian community also operated schools for its children.[4]

Said bin Taimur, sultan from 1932 to 1970, was educated in India. He adopted a reform program in the 1930s but, because of the curtailment of trade resulting from the Depression and the consequent decline of royal revenues, lacked the resources necessary to implement it. Because of an internal struggle for power in the 1950s, in which the sultan repressed opponents allied with Egypt and Saudi Arabia, there were few signs of advancements in health in that decade. Oil exploration crews created truck routes and roads in some areas in 1955 and thereafter, opening communication with parts of the interior. Muscat built water and sewerage systems. A development department, organized in 1959 and deploying some British resources, sought to expand health and education facilities and to improve agriculture and transport.[5] But Said, believing that general education would open Oman to Arab nationalism and threaten his power, supported only the two official primary schools at Muttrah and Salalah that trained young men for government service.

The United Nations made the first estimate of life expectancy in Oman, assessing it at 36.4 years in the early 1950s, a time when there was practically no information about mortality and even the population size was a matter of uncertainty.[6] If reliable, that is a high enough level to suggest that gains had already begun. Estimates of pre-transition life expectancy are available for three other countries in the region: Kuwait at 26 in the early years of the century, Iran at 25 in 1926, and Algeria at 28.8

in the 1920s. If conditions in Oman were similar for the same period, then as much as 8 to 10 years might have been added to life expectancy in the 1940s and very early 1950s. But, as noted, the descriptive evidence seems to be at odds with a picture of such a pace of gains. That is true also of the 1950s. UN estimates suggest improvement from 36.4 years in the early 1950s to 41.3 in the early 1960s, a pace of 0.5 years advance per year of calendar time, which, again, the descriptive evidence does not support.

Both the United Nations Development Program and the World Bank maintain that Omani life expectancy rose sharply during the 1960s, and for the first time there are several positive developments in harmony with such a claim.[7] Oil exploration had begun in the 1920s, but commercial quantities of oil were not found until 1964. After construction of a pipeline from Fahud to Muscat, production and exports began in 1967. A 1962 proposal that Oman should join the World Health Organization (WHO), and thereby qualify for its programs, was opposed by the Soviet Union and the United Arab Republic and was therefore deferred.[8] Nevertheless, programs of social development were introduced, more roads were built, and about twenty health centers were opened around the country (most earlier development had been concentrated in the coastal area) along with a mobile medical service for pastoralists; the clinics and mobile service were staffed chiefly by male nurses from India.[9] Survival in urban areas came unmistakably to surpass that in the countryside, so that rising life expectancy in Oman was assisted by urbanization: the proportion of the population living in urban areas rose from 4 percent cent in 1960 to 72 percent by 2000.

Ian Skeet, who worked in Oman between 1966 and 1968 for a British company, described the country in detail and gives less reason to suppose that survival was improving so rapidly. In Muscat, the capital, only the elite enjoyed piped water; others were served by wells or by daily deliveries carried by donkeys or men. In nearby Muttrah, the commercial center and the largest city in the country, the beachfront served as public toilet, and the town lacked sanitary facilities for the disposal of human waste or refuse. The diseases of poverty were still common. Skeet saw great potential for development, but, like Western visitors for several centuries, he noticed most the signs of underdevelopment and wrote of development as something lying ahead: "What Omanis yearn for most of all is the opportunity to educate their children."[10] Given such descriptions and the fact that oil revenues fed rising GDP only from 1967, the UN life expectancy estimates still seem to locate survival gains implausibly, at the leading edge of investments in health, and to suggest that oil revenues were almost immediately brought to bear in ways productive of better health.

Said's son, Qaboos, who was educated in Britain, deposed his father in July 1970 and, with British and U.S. support and advice from foreign experts, quickly adopted a broad program of medical, social, and economic development while keeping autocratic power, even after the adoption of a constitution in 1996. If the potential explanations for gains in life expectancy before 1970 are too few and often also too vague, the explanations for the period after 1970 are numerous and specific. Omani exiles, some of them holding professional degrees, returned as job opportunities opened for them in the more progressive regime. The new Ministry of Health promoted vaccination, clinics, piped water, swamp drainage, and anti-mosquito spraying. It also provided health education, especially for female students, plus child care classes for adult women, and hired physicians and nurses from abroad. Schooling expanded quickly; the mere 900 students, all male, enrolled in 1970 grew to 35,565 students, still mostly boys, in 1973–74, and to 474,937 students, with nearly equal numbers of males and females, in 1994–95. Trachoma prevalence plunged from 95 percent of the populace in the early 1970s to 5 percent in the late 1980s.[11]

Oman stands nearly alone in the pace at which it added to survival in the 1970s and early 1980s, peaking at a gain of 1.6 years per year of calendar time in the late 1970s.[12] Oil revenues, comprising 96 percent of government income in the 1970s, made it possible to invest in health. But the most striking feature of Oman's health transition is the comparatively modest size of the per capita spending on health-related items, which Allan Hill and Lincoln Chen estimate at $138 in 1994, much below the level in high-income countries at that time.[13] Qaboos Bin Said thus shared these oil revenues with his subjects by quickly building a health infrastructure featuring hospitals, health centers, maternity clinics, and outpatient centers (some mobile for the rural populace made up mostly of subsistence farmers), and a medical school; by investing in the standard of living via subsidized housing for low income families; and by providing free public education at all levels.[14] In 1970 about 80 percent of the populace could not read and write, with the highest proportions among older people. The 1988–89 Child Health Survey found more than half of males at ages 45–49 and above illiterate, as were more than half of females at ages 25–29 and up.[15] Nevertheless, "the survival chances of children born to mothers with little or no education improved more rapidly than those of literate mothers."[16] In Oman nearly universal access to health care seems to have made enough of an impact to reduce the advantages conveyed to mothers by education. That is, the Oman system was good enough to render it unnecessary for women to need to possess the attributes associated with education in order to protect their children's health.

By 2002 Oman's life expectancy had reached 72.7, according to the UN estimate, or 74.1 according to the World Bank's World Development Indicators. In 2001 WHO ranked Oman's health system as the most efficient in the world. With its oil revenues, "Oman could have been wealthy but unhealthy." Instead Qaboos Bin Said used oil revenues to build a welfare state with a leading health sector. Investments in public health and medicine developed more or less parallel to one another and led the post-1970 gains in survival, but health services of good quality and easy access take the leading place in the Hill and Chen analysis.[17] Investments in those services became possible because of rapidly rising oil revenues, assisted by fortuitous timing: the 1975 oil shock delivered much higher revenues than had been anticipated.

As noted, the earlier gains remain incompletely understood; innovations before 1970 do not seem to have been extensive enough to account for the survival gains estimated by the United Nations. But if the assumption is then made that these gains were actually deferred until after 1970, the post-1970 pace will have been about twice as rapid as the already high pace indicated by estimates from the United Nations and Oman itself.[18] Allan Hill, A. Z. Muyeed, and J. A. al-Lawati discuss most changes in health services from the baseline of the government's first five-year plan, inaugurated in 1976.[19] That compresses the time available for such vast changes yet further.

The Oman case study has a number of important implications. It suggests that autocratic direction can, with adequate resources used efficiently, quickly elevate life expectancy. It is not necessary to invest in education, behavior change, and maternal and child health care training and then wait for those things to pay off. Instead a country untroubled by scarce resources can invest in public health and medicine and, even in the poor health conditions that prevailed in Oman in the 1950s, expect immediate and huge returns. The concentration of a population in urban areas, where medical and public health resources are most numerous, also helps. It seems likely, had individuals rather than the sultan made choices about spending, that less would have been done to improve housing, build schools and hire teachers, or construct elaborate and modern public health and medical sectors. It is surprising, even astonishing, that such efficient systems for delivering public health and medical services could be designed and built so quickly. Especially from the description given by Hill and Chen, Oman appears to have speedily built a health system that is far more efficient, as gauged by the levels of life expectancy and spending on health, than what is found in any of the high-income countries.

Other Cases in the Middle East and North Africa

Oman's efficiency in adding health services in the 1970s may well have been made possible by earlier developments in Kuwait.[20] Commercial deposits of oil were discovered there in 1938, but it was 1946, after World War II, before they could be developed into sizable exports. By the early 1950s Kuwait was earning substantial revenues from those exports and had begun a program of simultaneous infrastructure and social development. (Figure 4d in chapter 1 shows Kuwait's exceptional status in 1950 as a high-income country.) At that time health services were available only to a few, and only about 4,600 students were enrolled in primary schools. Much of the early 1950s investment was lost to corruption on the part of British companies holding construction contracts, and too often Kuwait bought costly medical equipment without having first established needs and priorities. By the late 1950s, however, Kuwait had expanded a small missionary health care program into an elaborate hospital-dominated system of services free to all, hiring physicians and nurses from abroad, often from Egypt. Oil revenues also subsidized housing, some foods, water and electricity, and pensions. Thus Kuwait pioneered a pattern in which oil revenues were shared with the general population in the form of health, educational, and social services and assistance in what Allan Hill terms a "welfare state system."[21] Kuwait achieved an early lead in life expectancy and life expectancy gains, and maintained it.

Some accounts of Oman's health investments in the 1970s emphasize the part played by foreign advisers in deciding what to do. But it may be that Kuwait's experience in the 1950s also proved an informative model, one that allowed the Omanis to avoid repeating the wasteful elements of Kuwait's early investments.

Figure 26 compares life expectancy change in Oman with that in Iran, Iraq, Kuwait, and Saudi Arabia.[22] UN estimates indicate a nearly parallel development among the five countries from the early 1950s through the early 1970s, but considerable disarray thereafter. Oman continued its gains, moving by the early 1980s to a trend line that essentially matched Saudi Arabia's. Wars temporarily compromised survival in Iran, Iraq, and Kuwait, and, in Iraq, the survival deficit associated with the post–Persian Gulf War embargo in the 1990s persisted to 2002.[23]

Compared to the others, Oman seems to have made the most effec-

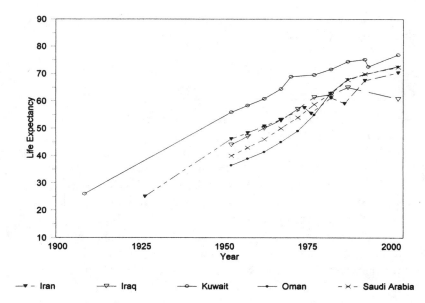

FIGURE 26. Life expectancy in Oman and four other Middle Eastern countries, 1900–2002.
SOURCES: United Nations, *Demographic Yearbook: Historical Supplement 1948–1997* CD-ROM (New York: Department of Economic and Social Affairs, Statistical Office, United Nations, n.d.); World Bank, *World Development Indicators 2004 on CD-ROM* (Washington: World Bank, 2004); also, Akbar Aghajanian, "Population Change in Iran 1966–86: A Stalled Demographic Transition?" *Population and Development Review* 17 (1991): 703–15; Allan G. Hill, "The Demography of the Kuwaiti Population of Kuwait," *Demography* 12 (1975): 537–48; and Hill and Lincoln C. Chen, *Oman's Leap to Good Health: A Summary of Rapid Health Transition in the Sultanate of Oman* (Muscat: n.p., 1996).

tive use of its oil revenues in the area of health. While Oman also built primary care facilities, it devoted a larger portion of spending to health centers for the rural population, in place of Kuwait's concentration of facilities in Kuwait City. According to UN estimates, all five countries enjoyed rapid gains in survival in the peaceful 1950s and 1960s.[24]

All five countries share some characteristics, including a pre-transition disease profile featuring many of the same diseases: malaria, tuberculosis, dengue, plague, cholera, yellow fever, trachoma, hookworm, fecal disease, typhoid fever, schistosomiasis, and typhus. In the pre-transition period they had few medical practitioners, hospital beds, or other facilities, but all subsequently invested heavily in building health services. Saudi Ara-

TABLE 12. Percentage of the Population Living in Urban Areas in 7 Countries, 1960–2002

	1960	1970	1980	1990	2002
Algeria	30	40	44	51	58
Iran	34	41	50	56	65
Iraq	43	56	66	70	67
Kuwait	72	78	91	95	96
Libya	23	46	69	80	86
Oman	4	11	32	62	77
Saudi Arabia	30	49	66	78	87

SOURCE: World Bank, World Development Indicators 2004 at devdata.worldbank.org/dataonline/SMResult.asp accessed November 4, 2004.

bia, in particular, followed the pattern of Kuwait: as oil revenues rose rapidly after World War II, Saudi Arabia made medicine the leading sector of investment. In 1949 the Saudi kingdom had about 111 physicians, in what may have been an early stage of survival gains, but the number grew to 1,172 by 1970 and 14,335 by 1985; many, as in Kuwait, were hired from Egypt. All these countries targeted certain diseases for control, including malaria and trachoma, often using DDT against mosquitoes. All recorded particularly rapid gains in infant and child survival. The rapid urbanization of the population also helped make it easier and more efficient to supply health services, education, and sanitary improvements. Table 12 shows, for the seven oil-rich Middle Eastern and North African countries, the proportion of the population living in urban areas for certain years of the period 1960–2002.

Figure 27 compares life expectancy in Algeria and Libya to that for Oman. Algeria's health transition may have begun years before the discovery of oil there in 1956, perhaps in the 1930s.[25] Both the slow gains of the 1930s and the very rapid postwar improvements that persisted up to the war of independence (1956–60) were therefore unrelated to oil revenues. However, Kamel Kateb's estimate of life expectancy, at 32.9 years for females and 33.9 for males in 1953–55, a peaceful period, is low enough to suggest that survival gains may not have begun until the 1950s or 1960s.[26] Certainly the bleak image that Yves Lacoste and André Prénant draw of public health, medical services, education, and economic conditions in the early 1950s allows little room to hypothesize about or to explain any prior gains.[27] In either case, investment in the health system led

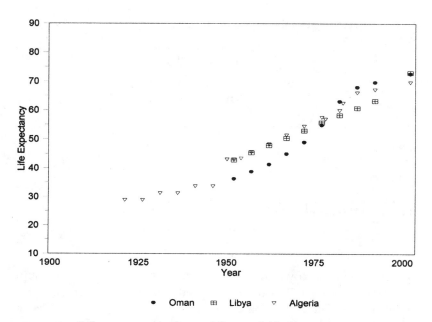

FIGURE 27. Life expectancy in Oman, Libya, and Algeria, 1900–2000.
SOURCES: Julien Condé, *Some Demographic Aspects of Human Resources in Africa* (Paris: Development Center of the Organization for Economic Cooperation and Development, 1973); United Nations, *Demographic Yearbook: Historical Supplement 1948–1997* CD-ROM (New York: Department of Economic and Social Affairs, Statistical Office, United Nations, n.d.); and World Bank, *World Development Indicators 2004 on CD-ROM* (Washington: World Bank, 2004).

to an "explosion" in medical facilities and personnel after independence in 1962 and, in the 1980s, rapid growth in the number of health centers and clinics.[28] In the mid-1960s more than two-thirds of Algerians were illiterate, but school enrollments were rising, along with the share of school-age girls who were attending school.[29]

Figure 28 compares changes in life expectancy and GDPpc in 1990 international dollars for Oman and Algeria, showing a rapid increase in Oman toward nearly $12,000, compared to fluctuation around $5,000 in Algeria, yet quite similar paths of survival gains. While Oman was an efficient provider of health services, Algeria was a still more efficient provider of factors that elevated life expectancy. This makes Algeria one of the most interesting cases for future study seeking to identify and weigh the importance of these factors.

In the case of Libya, oil exports began in 1961, at a point when life ex-

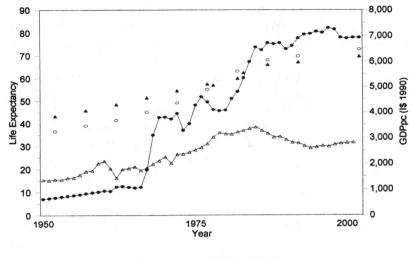

FIGURE 28. Gross domestic product per capita (GDPpc) in 1990 international dollars (I$) and life expectancy in Algeria and Oman, 1950–2000.
SOURCES: Julien Condé, *Some Demographic Aspects of Human Resources in Africa* (Paris: Development Center of the Organization for Economic Cooperation and Development, 1973); Allan G. Hill and Lincoln C. Chen, *Oman's Leap to Good Health: A Summary of Rapid Health Transition in the Sultanate of Oman* (Muscat: n.p., 1996); Angus Maddison, *The World Economy: Historical Statistics* (Paris: Development Center of the Organization for Economic Cooperation and Development, 2003), pp. 186–87, 218; United Nations, *Demographic Yearbook: Historical Supplement 1948–1997* CD-ROM (New York: Department of Economic and Social Affairs, Statistical Office, United Nations, n.d.); and World Bank, *World Development Indicators 2004 on CD-ROM* (Washington: World Bank, 2004)

pectancy at birth already was 47 or 48 years.[30] Most oil revenues were earmarked for economic and social development. Like the other oil-rich states considered here, Libya invested in medical personnel and hospitals and, somewhat later, in dispensaries.[31] Those investments were made before governing authorities knew much about either the level of mortality or causes of death. Since most physicians in the new system were hired from the outside, it can also be said that this system was constructed at a point when even medical personnel had an incomplete grasp of which diseases would be the most troublesome.

Most of the schooling available earlier had been in Islamic schools or, during the Italian colonial period, which began in 1911, for Italians. The British began building an educational system during the wartime period of their military government, and by 1950–51 some 33,000 students, mostly boys, were enrolled in various types of schools. Enrollments increased some during the 1950s, but it was the commercial exploitation of oil that provided Libya with the resources needed to expand schooling. By 1968–69 about 271,000 boys and girls were enrolled in elementary schools, and the central government was allocating the exceptionally high proportion of 24 percent of all spending to education. Teacher training facilities were added apace.[32]

Up to the revolution of 1969 that deposed him, King Idris operated a corrupt regime, yet one that also invested in health and education. And after Mu'ammar Gadhafi seized power in 1969, that investment was even higher.[33] Nonetheless, it appears that Libyan authorities set out to build the facilities for schooling and health care out of a general expectation that money should be spent in this way rather than because they had formulated specific objectives for the schools or clinics.

Venezuela

Venezuela created a variety of medical and public health institutions and organizations in the nineteenth century, including the Oficina de Sanidad Naciónal (OSN), but there is little in the record to suggest that any of these had an impact on the mortality level. (Venezuela will also be discussed in chapter 9, where income statistics appear in figures 32 and 33 and life expectancy estimates in table 13.) For such an impact the decisive factor was evidently the commercial production of oil that began in 1918, which provided the central state with revenues on a scale sufficient to invest in sanitation, public health, and education.[34] The OSN was spending about a half million bolívares in fiscal year 1911–12; this jumped by 1929–30 to 3.5 million.[35] Life expectancy began to improve in a persistent way in Venezuela in the 1920s or 1930s.

Following Spanish usage, the Venezuelan government claimed subsurface mineral wealth. Oil exploitation was turned over to foreign companies in return for fees, royalties, and tax revenues, which delivered vast new resources. Government revenues rose sharply between 1918 and 1930 and again from 1942 to 1954, with the Venezuelan congress typically extracting better terms from producers than had Juan Vicente Gómez, the dictator who died in 1935.[36] By 1929 more than half of Venezuela's public sector expenditures were allocated to economic and social development.[37] Throughout this period Venezuela allocated a larger share of its revenues to economic than to social investments, more to roads, railroads, irrigation and agricultural development, and public works than to schools, medical improvements, or public health facilities even if spending on water and drainage facilities are grouped as health expenditures. Most of the scholarly attention given Venezuela's development path has concentrated on economic development, and most researchers have expressed disappointment about Venezuela's progress.[38] Was social development equally disappointing?

Malaria was widespread in the early twentieth century, with about half the population being infected.[39] Arturo Luis Bertí and José Antonio Jove trace public health activism to 1924 and the campaign against malaria organized by the OSN that year.[40] Venezuela reached an agreement with the Rockefeller Foundation to conduct surveys of hookworm and malaria in 1926, and in 1927 initiated a campaign against hookworm in the Maracay region, building latrines, treating infected people, and indoctrinating the public in the dangers of hookworm and of the fecal disease associated with it, which could be prevented by the safe disposal of human waste. In the meantime both the government and foreign oil companies invested in health and education facilities for oil workers and other people living in the Lake Maracaibo area. A campaign against malaria relying heavily on the larvicide Paris green and oil spraying was begun about the same time in regions of the country where the disease was a problem. By 1932 Venezuela was producing its own BCG vaccine for use against tuberculosis. The Rockefeller Foundation withdrew in 1933, but work against all three diseases was pursued through the 1930s and 1940s.[41] In Caracas, where the construction of water and sewage facilities made good headway in the 1930s, infant mortality dropped in the period 1928–35.[42]

Social development spending rose faster from 1936 under the Ministerio de Sanidad y Asistencia Social (MSAS), and more rapidly still from 1943, when oil revenues surged. In the late 1930s MSAS spending averaged 5.5 percent of government expenditures; after 1943 that increased to an average closer to 7 percent even as the spending total also increased. (This share is low compared to what Mexico was already spending on social development in all forms, but much higher than earlier spending levels in Venezuela.) Especially between 1943 and 1949 the government built clinics in rural areas and staffed them with physicians; in the same decade the government began building water and drainage facilities for rural towns.[43] Medical facilities, especially for tertiary care, remained concentrated in Caracas and the other cities. Venezuela also built primary schools, created more spaces for children to attend schools, and trained teachers in new normal schools. By 1950 primary school enrollment had risen more than tenfold over the 1917 level.[44] The 1941 census indicated that some 57 percent of people aged 10 and above were illiterate; by 1971 the number had dropped to 23 percent.

These investments put Venezuela in the lead in South America in building a health infrastructure. Pan American Health Organization estimates for 1969 show the country far ahead of its neighbors in providing safe water in urban and rural areas, and a leader in the safe disposal of human waste.[45]

Although campaigns were mounted against other diseases as well, Venezuela persisted in trying to control fecal disease, malaria, and tuberculosis, which had been leading causes of death. In 1945, DDT succeeded Paris green as the chief chemical weapon against anopheles mosquitoes, and its use continued through the mid-1950s. José Avilán and colleagues identify gastrointestinal diseases as the leading cause of death in 1940–44, with tuberculosis second, and malaria fourth. By 1963–67 malaria had become a minor cause of death; gastrointestinal diseases had dropped to fifth and tuberculosis to ninth place among causes of death.[46]

In the long run, urbanization proved an ally because it was easier to control many leading diseases in urban than in rural areas. About 15 percent of the Venezuelan population lived in cities in 1926. That proportion rose to 29 percent in 1936, about 50 percent in 1950, 61 percent in 1960, and by 2002 to 87 percent. Like the oil-rich states of the Middle East and North Africa, Venezuela benefited from urbanization, but movement into cities developed earlier in Venezuela than in most of the others.

Conclusion

Observers have termed some of the oil-rich states considered here examples of state socialism, but the term fits poorly. It is true that these oil states provided services and benefits in the form of socialism by investing in medicine, public health, and education, and some of them also in housing and a minimum living standard. But the decisions to do that were usually made in a paternalistic fashion, without asking people how they might have preferred to have the oil riches spent and without developing an ideology favoring the democratization of these services. Thus the notion of "oil paternalism" better captures this scheme.

But the important point is that oil wealth was spent to the benefit of population health—in Venezuela from the 1920s under the dictator Gómez (although more generously by his successors, after his death in 1935, and in periods of democratic governance), and later in Algeria, Libya, Oman, and Saudi Arabia. In each case these autocrats spent a great deal on themselves, their families, and their entourages, giving rise to a valid international picture of selfish indulgence. But they also spent on their people, and that the spending had good effects in the area of survival.

The oil-rich countries in the Middle East and North Africa, with the possible exception of Oman, seem to have been cases where vast new financial resources were thrown at the problem of poor population health with little advance planning or understanding of how to use those resources efficiently. Nevertheless, none are cases of failure. All of these lands invested in health facilities and broad access to health care. Given their especially rapid gains in survival, these countries seem to provide the best examples of pay-offs from a concentration on medicine in the form of wide access to health care. True, schools and education were also emphasized, but it is unrealistic to expect those effects to have been immediate. None of these countries invested as heavily in public health, but they did build public health amenities in major cities, including water and sewage systems, so that progress in survival was assisted both by these facilities and by urbanization. Perhaps the most remarkable feature of these seven countries, however, is that they made rapid progress in survival by investing more in medicine than they had earlier done, but still investing at levels that left them far behind per capita spending on health care in the high-income lands.

In the West social spending came to prominence in the period 1850–1930, when governments began to invest more heavily in education, public health, the provision of such medical facilities as hospitals and dispensaries, training of nurses and doctors, pensions, health insurance, and other areas. Peter Lindert argues that social spending did not really develop before about 1880, and when it did, its expansion was initially due, in the Western countries he considered, to open and democratic political regimes, population aging, and Protestantism.[47] Venezuela came later to new social initiatives, and the oil-rich states of the Middle East and North Africa later still. They invested in quite similar ways, and at times in history when higher investments in education, medical facilities and personnel, and public health could pay more immediate and more efficient benefits. All of them made these investments much more from the rulers' sense of what the people needed than from any expression by the people of what they wanted. But it is also true that social spending increased more in

Venezuela in periods of representative government than in periods of dictatorship.

Up to the case of Oman in the 1970s and 1980s, the oil-rich countries of the Middle East and North Africa seem to have been instances of inefficient despotism. Autocrats and rulers who governed without popular participation made decisions that benefited population health, plunging suddenly into massive spending, much of it wasteful. They spent simultaneously on medicine, public health, and education and, despite the inefficiency, the investments paid off in almost immediate gains in survival at a pace as high as attained anywhere in any period. By comparison, Venezuela used its oil revenues to promote both economic and social development but had greater success in the latter.

Some newer oil-rich states, including Nigeria and Equatorial Guinea, have not followed the same path. Nigeria invested in roads and, to a lesser degree, in schools, but in both of these countries vast revenues from oil disappeared, apparently into the pockets of members of the regime and their cronies, with little new investment in public health or medicine and a continuing poor record in survival.

CHAPTER 9

The Latin American Case

Income Inequality and Health in Mexico

Countries with marked inequality in the distribution of income or wealth may find it difficult to elevate life expectancy. According to G. B. Rodgers, a more even distribution of income and wealth gives more households an opportunity to acquire goods and services that may positively influence survival, such as more spacious housing, household amenities including piped water and indoor plumbing, health care, more years of schooling for parents or children, electricity and refrigerators, and so forth.[1] On the face of this argument, the Latin American countries of Mexico, Argentina, Chile, and Uruguay—but especially Mexico and Chile, which for a long time were much poorer than Argentina or Uruguay—might be expected to have faced serious difficulties in elevating life expectancy.

Table 13 shows the development of life expectancy in these four countries, plus Venezuela, discussed in chapter 8. According to official crude death rate statistics, which exclude the indigenous population and may understate mortality, Uruguay was one of the healthiest countries in the world in the latter part of the nineteenth century but made slow progress in survival gains until the 1930s and 1940s.[2] Argentina, in contrast, began a long phase of rapid gains around 1900, catching up to official estimates for Uruguay in the 1920s. Both were precocious in economic development, although their early successes did not translate into sustained economic growth. Mexico and Chile, along with Venezuela, lagged behind in life expectancy until the 1960s. Mexico initiated a health transition in the latter part of the nineteenth century from an unusually low level of survival in the early nineteenth century; Chilean survival began to improve in the 1920s; Venezuela's health transition

TABLE 13. Life Expectancy in 5 Countries in Latin America, 1875–2000

	1875	1900	1925	1950	1975	2000
Argentina	33.2	35.1	51.4	62.0	68.2	73.9
Chile	30.2	32.7	34.3	51.2	65.7	75.7
Mexico	n.a.	27.6	32.1	49.6	64.3	73.0
Uruguay	n.a.	n.a.	53.6	61.3	69.0	74.4
Venezuela	30	n.a.	34	53.9	67.0	73.4

SOURCES: *For Argentina:* Héctor Pérez Brignoli, *El crecimiento demográfico de America Latina en los siglos XIX y XX: Problemas, metodos y perspectives* (San José: Centro de Investigaciónes Historicas, Universidad de Costa Rica, 1989), p. 13; Jorge L. Somoza, *La Mortalidad en la Argentina entre 1869 y 1960* (Buenos Aires: Instituto Torcuato di Tella, Editorial del Instituto, 1971), esp. pp. 19, 26, 28; Somoza, "La Mortalidad en la Argentina entre 1869 y 1960," *Desarrollo económico* 12 (1973): 807–26; and United Nations, *Demographic Yearbook: Historical Supplement 1948–1997* CD-ROM (New York: Department of Economic and Social Affairs, Statistical Office, United Nations, n.d.). *For Chile:* Pérez Brignoli, *El crecimiento demográfico de America Latina,* p. 13; and World Bank, *World Development Indicators 2004 on CD-ROM* (Washington: World Bank, 2004). *For Mexico:* Eduardo E. Arriaga, *New Life Tables for Latin American Populations in the Nineteenth and Twentieth Centuries* (Berkeley: University of California Press, 1968), p. 170–75, 198–207; M. A. Bravo Becherelle and R. Jiménez Reyes, "Tablas de vida para México 1893 a 1956," *Revista del Instituto de Salubridad y Enfermedades Tropicales* 18 (1958): 81–136; Sergio Camposortega Cruz, *Análisis demográfico de la mortalidad en México, 1940–1980* (Mexico City: Centro de Estudios Demográficos y de Desarrollo Urbano, Colegio de México, 1992); and Pérez Brignoli, *El crecimiento demográfico de America Latina,* p. 14, reporting results derived by Mier y Terán and Collver. *For Uruguay:* Américo Migliónico, *La Mortalidad en Uruguay en el siglo XX: Cambios, impacto, perpectivas* (Montevideo: Ministerio de Salud Público, 2001); Migliónico, *Tablas abreviadas de mortalidad por sexo y edad: Total del país, 1908 a 1999* (Montevideo: Ministerio de Salud Público, 2001); and World Bank, *World Development Indicators 2004. For Venezuela:* Chi-Yi Chen and Michel Picouet, *Dinámica de la población: Caso de Venezuela* (Caracas: Edición UCAB-ORSTROM, 1979), p. 33; and United Nations, *Demographic Yearbook: Historical Supplement 1948–1997.*

(as we have already seen) began in the 1920s or 1930s. Mexico, Chile, and Venezuela made especially rapid gains between 1920 and the 1960s, and by 1970 closed most of the gap separating them from Argentina and Uruguay.

Figure 29 compares Maddison's estimates of GDPpc in these five countries in 1990 international dollars (I$). Argentina achieved a GDPpc level above I$ 2,000 before 1900, as did Uruguay, while Chile as well as Mexico and Venezuela lagged. Venezuela's exceptional oil wealth shows up in the rapid rise of per capita income from 1920 to about 1960. By the 1990s all five countries could be classified as middle-income. Because of this, their achievements in life expectancy may seem less impressive. What is more important to notice, however, is that all five initiated sustained gains in survival from low-income positions and made strong gains in survival well before attaining the position of a middle-income country *and* without altering their longstanding unequal distribution of income.[3]

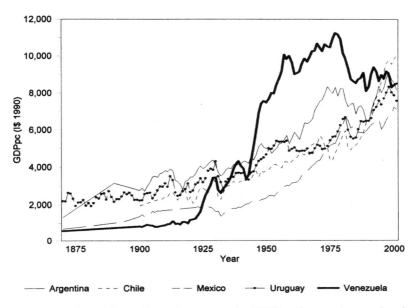

FIGURE 29. Gross domestic product per capita (GPDpc) in 1990 international dollars (I$) in five Latin American countries, 1870–2000.
SOURCE: Angus Maddison, *The World Economy: Historical Statistics* (Paris: Development Center of the Organization for Economic Cooperation and Development, 2003), pp. 142–44.

Figure 30 shows estimates of the Gini coefficient for the distribution of household income in these five countries, plus Sweden, in the period 1950–2000. Mexico and Chile both averaged 0.54, Venezuela 0.45, Argentina 0.42, and Uruguay 0.34, compared to Sweden's average in the same period of 0.22. The higher numbers identify countries where elites claimed a disproportionately large share of income—and indeed in Latin America this distribution is and has long been as unequal as in any world region.[4] Thus the GDPpc averages mask quite substantially lower average incomes in the bottom half of households, especially in Mexico and Chile, and much higher average incomes in the top 10 or 20 percent of households.

What matters most, as Rodgers argues, is what income distribution suggests about the capacity of households in the bottom half to afford investments that pay health dividends. In a society with a more egalitarian distribution, where lower income households share in gains, periods of income growth provide an opportunity to make such investments. But in skew distributions that is less likely to happen. There it may be neces-

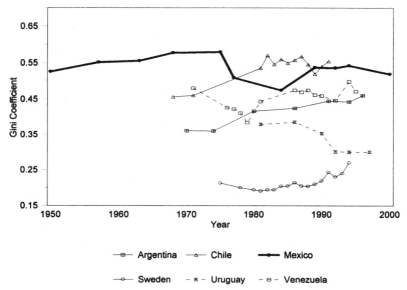

FIGURE 30. Inequality in income distribution in five Latin American countries and Sweden, 1950–2000, by Gini coefficient.
SOURCES: Anders Björklund and Mårten Palme, "The Evolution of Income Inequality during the Rise of the Swedish Welfare State 1951 to 1973," *Nordic Journal of Political Economy* 26 (2000): 115–28; Samuel Morley, *The Income Distribution Problem in Latin America and the Caribbean* (Santiago: ECLAC, 2001), pp. 166–69; and the United Nations Development Programme World Income Inequality Database at http://www.wider.unu.edu/wiid/wwwwiid .htm, accessed 3/24/2005.

sary, if such investments are to be made, for government spending to lead the way in making them.

Mexico is thus the most interesting case study here because it faced two problems: the lowest level of per capita income in this group of Latin American countries, and, for most of this period, the distribution of income most skewed toward the elite. These combined to leave poor families with extremely limited resources.

Mexico's Investment in Education

Zadia Feliciano attributes survival gains in the 1920s and 1930s especially to economic growth and to the opportunity that rising incomes gave Mexicans "to buy more food, better housing and more health care."[5] But Mexico was a mostly rural country where people in the countryside, especially Indians, lived in profound poverty and isolation from the economic growth associated with foreign trade and the development of oil. (Because revenues were more modest per capita, oil played a smaller part in government revenues and overall economic activity in Mexico than in the oil-rich states discussed in chapter 8.) The key elements of an account of survival gains in Mexico must therefore deal with changes in rural areas.

Nineteenth-century Mexico was a profoundly inegalitarian society in which a small group of landowners and urban elites claimed shares of income, wealth, and political power that vastly surpassed their portion of the population. The idea that these circumstances should change motivated many participants in the Mexican Revolution of 1910–20 and their cry for "land and liberty." The Constitution of 1917 promised fundamental reforms, including land redistribution, which remained the actual objectives of reformists into the 1940s and rhetorical objectives of political leaders into the 1980s. The constitution set an ambitious agenda, parts of which were realized in the 1920s and 1930s.

Miguel Bustamante reports causes of death in the period 1922–33 using official data, which underreport deaths and also give causes for only a portion of the deaths reported. According to these incomplete records, the leading reported cause of death was the group of fecal or gastrointestinal diseases: diarrhea and enteritis, dysentery, and typhoid fever. Fever, without further identification, malaria, and tuberculosis also caused many deaths; along with pneumonia and smallpox these were the leading causes in a profile that closely resembled that faced in Jamaica and Venezuela in the same period.[6]

Mexican leaders concerned with improving population health, including President Alvaro Obregón, who served from 1920 to 1924, believed that spreading education and literacy in a mostly illiterate land could lead to better health and teach children personal hygiene.[7] Pre-revolutionary education had aimed to school the elite to a European standard. Revolutionary aims added rural schooling and education for the poor to a minimum standard having less to do with literacy than with imparting certain useful information: "primary stress was placed on changing the [social] environment rather than on eliminating the high percentage of illiteracy."[8] About 80 percent of adults were illiterate in 1910, and few people in a mostly rural nation had any contact with educated people or printed material.

José Vasconcelos, the inaugural secretary of education in the department organized in 1921, formulated a plan to promote cultural missions and another to build rural schools, train teachers in normal schools in rural areas, and produce school materials, which he and his successors carried out. The cultural missions consisted of people with specialized knowledge who traveled from one rural locale to another teaching what they knew, including hygiene, reading, nationalism, and useful skills. From 1926 these *misioneros* were trained more specifically in sanitation and community work so that they would teach about sanitation and the germ theory of disease. They showed peasants how to build privies and wells that provided safe water, explained techniques of sanitary cooking, and provided information about specific diseases, including malaria and tuberculosis, and how to combat them. Thousands of new schools, in rural areas called *casas del pueblo,* were built, mostly at local expense, while the national government paid for school materials and teachers. In the evenings the schools were used for adult education, including a public health campaign and lessons in child care. Progress in building schools and enrolling students was particularly rapid from the take-off period of 1925–28, when enrollments passed their pre-revolutionary level.[9] Public sector spending on education jumped in 1931 to 13 percent of overall spending and for several decades thereafter remained within the unusually high range of 7–14 percent.[10]

By 1928 schools were using primers that featured material about hygiene, in part because Vasconcelos wanted in particular to persuade peasants to bathe regularly.[11] And in the 1930s the Secretaría de Educación Pública distributed material aimed at teachers that featured explanations about how to build latrines and improve diet quality. Schoolteachers, many of them women, learned to give smallpox vaccinations and led campaigns promoting village and household cleanliness.[12] James Angus McLeod describes the teachers as public health aides on a model copied widely in Latin America afterwards.[13]

In some other countries higher investments in education paid off in rising school enrollments, female attendance that surpassed male attendance, and higher literacy. Mexico made some improvements in these areas while retaining its system for educating the elite to a European standard. But literacy in Spanish advanced slowly, mostly behind the improvement of survival. The disabilities that rural, non–Spanish speaking groups and women faced in competing for wealth, jobs, political power, and other markers of status persisted. Women first voted in national elections in 1955 but, especially in lower income households, "women's economic position remain[ed] constrained" much longer by the idea that their primary roles should be as wives and mothers.[14] Thus the changes that occurred in Mexico between 1920 and 1950 had little to do with a more democratic sharing of resources or with an improved status for women, and more to do with the mastery by rural peasants of information useful for controlling health risks and with higher public investments in education and public health.

Mexico's Investment in Public Health

The constitution of 1917 also made public health a responsibility of the state, and public sector spending in that area rose accordingly.[15] Some other practical steps toward addressing this promise were taken by agents of the Rockefeller Foundation, who initiated a campaign against yellow fever in 1920 and in 1924 mounted a campaign against hookworm. (At that time it was not an uncommon sight to see Mexicans "defecating in the principal streets of the smaller towns.") Foundation agents promoted the building and use of pit latrines.[16] In 1927 the Foundation and the Mexican Health Department began to work together to build rural sanitary units, which promoted latrine building, in some regions. Mortality from infectious, parasitic, and respiratory diseases declined, as did deaths from accidents and violence.[17]

Improvements in rural health care date mostly from the 1930s, when the *Nicolaitas,* a private group of socialist physicians inspired by changes proposed in the Soviet Union, led an effort to organize clinics and to staff them with medical students willing to serve in the countryside. Beginning in the vicinity of Morelia, these clinics were established on the *ejidos,* or agricultural cooperatives, that claimed an expanding share of land under cultivation. "The *Nicolaitas* regarded public health programs as a form of wealth redistribution," although they have been criticized for approaching the problem of providing health care and instructing peasants in sanitation in ways that disparaged the people they intended to assist. At the movement's peak, around 1941, 120 rural medical units were providing health care to some 300,000 people. But with the end of the presidency of Lázaro Cárdenas, who while in office from 1934 to 1940 had made rural health a matter of special concern, the program slowly withered to only those areas whose peasants could afford to shoulder the cost.[18] Overall, public spending on social welfare rose sharply from 1920 to 1940, stagnated during 1941–58, and after that increased again.[19]

Public works projects in the period 1890–1910 provided wealthier neighborhoods in Mexico City and some other urban locales with safe water and sewage disposal. But sanitary improvements of these types made little headway among the urban poor or in rural areas then or in the 1920s and 1930s.[20] Many small towns acquired potable water systems, but villages did not. Vaccinations reduced mortality from smallpox and perhaps also from typhoid fever, and malaria mortality decreased abruptly between 1935 and 1940 as a result of mosquito control porgrams.[21]

Infant mortality remained higher in rural than urban regions across the period 1940–60.[22] As late as 1960, 80 percent of dwellings in the country had one or two rooms, and only a minority, sometimes a small minority, had piped water or indoor plumbing. Nor did economic growth improve the distribution of income across households or regions even though, from 1940 to 1970, the economy grew at an impressive pace of about 6 percent a year. Thus none of the activities discussed above removed, or even much reduced, inequalities and unevenness across the land, and especially between urban and rural areas, in schooling, access to health care, potable water, mortality, and other health indicators. As of the 1970s, as James Horn argues, the egalitarian goals of the Mexican Revolution had not been achieved in health or health care.[23] Profound socioeconomic and regional disparities remained in place in Mexico in the 1980s and 1990s.[24] Nevertheless Mexico had by the mid-1970s attained a life expectancy at birth of 64 years. Although whole regions of the country had not closed the gaps in social development or in income, they had kept pace with favored groups in the society. Thus Mexico achieved high life expectancy, moving above 70 years in about 1990, without making fundamental changes in the structural inequalities that had existed before the beginning of its health transition.

Conclusion

In many Latin American countries an unequal distribution of income prevailed across the entire period of gains in survival. As has been noted, lower-income households have less opportunity to acquire goods and services that improve health, and uneven distribution could have weighed heavily against survival gains. But several countries in the region rose into a middle-income position and moved rapidly to converge with countries leading in life expectancy while retaining income distributions among the most uneven to be found around the world.

What happened, at least in Mexico and Venezuela, was that the public sector's social spending supplied some critical factors directly to house-holds. More especially in Mexico, but to some degree also in Venezuela, social spending developed in a paternalistic way. Even though the Mexican Revolution of 1910–20 is usually interpreted as an expression of popular discontent with a class-ridden society and polity, the reforms implemented in the 1920s and 1930s came mostly from above. Government investments in education and public health, and higher social spending in general, responded to the needs of an impoverished populace without specific programs having been influenced by the popular will. Venezuela had enough additional resources from oil to fund its projects in social development. But Mexico, whose oil revenues were much smaller, relied more on social missionaries, teachers who acted as health aides, and the willingness of the rural poor to be directed and led by these urban cadres.

CHAPTER 10

Limiting Mortality from Fecal Disease, Malaria, and Tuberculosis

Disease plays the central role in the history of human longevity. In the case studies of survival assembled here the three most important diseases have been the complex including dysentery, typhoid fever, and other unspecified diarrhea, which share the characteristic of being communicated in human fecal matter; malaria; and pulmonary tuberculosis. Because these diseases accounted for such a large share of deaths, significant gains in survival were difficult to achieve without reducing mortality from one or more of the three. This chapter brings together explanations of how mortality from these diseases was reduced in the period 1920–45, before the availability of DDT, which proved so powerful in controlling mosquito populations and therefore in reducing malaria mortality, and before the introduction of the antibiotics that made it possible to treat and cure typhoid fever and some other diarrheal diseases, and to treat and manage tuberculosis.

Fecal disease kills some people at every age, but the diseases transmitted in human waste have had their most profound impact on infants, children, youths, and young adults up to age 30 or so. Infants and young children often died during bouts of diarrhea of unspecific origin; typhoid fever caused many deaths in youth and young adulthood. Malaria, too, killed people of all ages, but most often infants and young children. Mortality from pulmonary tuberculosis, far and away the leading form of tuberculosis, peaked in young adulthood but was also common in later childhood, especially among girls.

Table 14 reports on eleven of the case-study countries, summarizing whether they reduced mortality from these diseases and when infant mor-

TABLE 14. Infant Mortality and Mortality from 3 Diseases in 11 Countries, 1920–1950

	Beginning of Decline in Infant Mortality	Decline in Mortality from Disease		
		Fecal Disease	*Malaria*	*Pulmonary Tuberculosis*
China	1920s or 1930s	uncertain	uncertain	uncertain
Costa Rica	1920s	yes	yes	yes
Cuba	1900s	yes	yes	yes
Jamaica	1920s	yes	yes	yes
Japan	1920s	cholera but not others	no information	declined 1919–33, rose 1933–45
Korea	1930s	uncertain	uncertain	probably not
Mexico	1920s	yes	yes	yes
Panama	1920s	yes	yes	no information
Russia	1920s	yes	from late 1930s	uncertain; in Moscow official statistics indicate mortality decline from c. 1900
Sri Lanka	1920s	yes	maybe	uncertain
Venezuela	1920s or 1930s	yes	yes	yes

SOURCES: Sources on mortality from the three diseases are given in the case studies and, in greater detail, in James C. Riley, "Bibliography of Works Providing Estimates of Life Expectancy at Birth and of the Beginning Period of Health Transitions in Countries with a Population in 2000 of at least 400,000" at www.lifetable.de/RileyBib.htm.

tality began to decline. (Oman is excluded from this table because its survival gains began after DDT, antibiotics, and other medical innovations became available.) In every case declining infant mortality, due in part to the control of malaria and fecal disease, may have been the greatest contributor to gains in life expectancy, but the gains also included improved survival at higher ages from two or all three of the diseases examined in this chapter.

Fecal Disease

Many different diseases may be transmitted in fecal matter, either directly, through contact with feces or eating or drinking contaminated water and foods, or indirectly, via fomites (contaminated items such as dishes or clothing), via worms excreted by carriers, or by flies and other insects that feed on fecal material. Most of the diseases transmitted in these ways have diarrhea as a symptom. People sick with cholera, typhoid and paratyphoid fever, amoebic and bacillary dysentery, and undifferentiated diarrhea excrete pathogens in their fecal matter during part or all of the period of sickness. The pathogens of some of these diseases are also excreted by apparently healthy carriers.[1]

Nearly everywhere in the world in the mid-nineteenth century people disposed of their fecal waste in ways that show they did not associate this waste with disease or disease transmission. Children defecated on the ground immediately surrounding rural housing or, in cities, at any convenient site out of doors. In Teheran in the 1920s League of Nations observers noticed that children defecated in the city's water supply without alarming anyone. At that time mosques furnished latrines for the men who prayed in them, but there were as yet no public latrines in the city. (The sources do not report where women defecated.) In villages and towns in Persia there were no sanitation facilities, and people prepared food heedless of houseflies.[2] Although practices began to change in the mid-nineteenth century in parts of the world, these conditions persisted in the countries considered here and allowed fecal disease to account for a large share of mortality, especially in infants and children.

As noted in the introduction, the filth theory of disease had associated general uncleanliness with sickness and, by the 1840s, pointed to fecal matter as an important category of filth. Thus urban elite and middle-class householders in Western Europe began in the mid-nineteenth century to replace cesspits with flush toilets and sewers, which evacuated waste matter from the household without having to use chamber pots or buckets and without having periodically to empty cesspits. By the end of the nineteenth century, the germ theory, prefigured most notably by Robert Koch's work on cholera in Egypt and India, in which he investigated fecal specimens, confirmed and explained the association between fecal matter and disease. The great era of sanitary improvements in Western cities then came in the period 1890 to 1930, when cities expanded systems to draw, filter, and chlorinate water, to pipe water into households, and then to remove wastewater, including the waterborne fecal matter, from households. Outside the Western world many cities built water and waste disposal systems for elite neighborhoods, but few managed to extend these systems to a majority of neighborhoods.

Such improvements simply exceeded what rural areas could afford.

Nevertheless a parallel but quite different series of improvements began in the same period in rural areas in which householders, alerted to the disease risks posed by fecal matter, distanced the places where they disposed of human waste from wells and streams and began to use pit latrines to capture feces. By the 1920s pit latrines might also incorporate features that reduced odor and blocked access by houseflies. In general, improvements in disposing of fecal matter began earlier in the cities and countryside in Western countries. But by the early twentieth century, and especially by the 1920s, cities and rural residents in Asia, Eastern Europe, and Latin America and the Caribbean were adopting inexpensive versions of these devices to reduce the contamination of water with feces and to dispose of fecal matter in ways that reduced chances of disease. Health authorities in many countries in Latin America, Asia, and Oceania promoted the use of pit latrines specifically as a way to reduce levels of infection from hookworm. In many countries latrine building was the key step recommended by Rockefeller Foundation agents, who worked in eighty countries to control hookworm and to limit what they called soil pollution (depositing feces on the surface of the ground) by inducing householders to build latrines. In some countries, these efforts succeeded—households built and used pit latrines, and public institutions, such as hospitals and schools, added latrines—while in others the anti-hookworm campaign accomplished little. Many countries in the same regions also introduced primary and middle school programs to educate children attending schools, and through them adults, about how they could recognize communicable diseases of importance, how those diseases were transmitted, and what simple and inexpensive steps people might take to protect themselves.

Jamaica's campaign remains the one most thoroughly studied, and a summary of its development can serve as an example of what a well-organized and persistent effort achieved. As discussed in chapter 6, the leading figure there was a Rockefeller agent, Benjamin Washburn, who remained in Jamaica from 1920 to 1937. British health authorities had been aware of hookworm as a disease before Washburn's arrival, but it was the resources provided by the Rockefeller Foundation that led to action. The main innovation of the 1910s was the addition of hygiene material to the primary school curriculum. Washburn set for himself the goal not of eradicating hookworm, which had been the initial yet unfulfilled hope of the anti-hookworm campaign elsewhere, but of developing the public health consciousness of the people, inducing them to develop new health-conscious behaviors and to become politically active in demanding better health programs from their local officials. In pursuit of those goals he organized two teams to move systematically from one parish to the next. The physician in each team "sounded" people, using a stethoscope to listen to their hearts; told people about hookworm; showed a silent film titled *Unhooking the Hookworm*; and in other ways demonstrated how hookworm infection occurred and explained the results of infection. Nurses moved house to house asking people to provide fecal specimens, microscopists examined the specimens to determine infection, and then the doctor and nurses treated and re-treated the infected, up to half a dozen times. Meanwhile team members told people how to avoid hookworm in the future by digging and using pit latrines. In one of the essays that he wrote for distribution in the monthly periodical *Jamaica Public Health,* Washburn explained the principles of waste disposal:

Another essential of health is that every home should have a safe means of getting rid of its sewage or bowel wastes. If there is no latrine, or only an open one, the soil becomes dirty from being mixed with bowel filth, and this is carried by flies to the food, or rains may wash it upon vegetables and it is eaten. This is the way most of the bowel filth diseases are spread. To stop this spread the bowel waste must be put where it cannot be scattered and where flies cannot reach it. This can be done by building a sanitary fly-tight latrine at each house and by the use of a latrine by every member of the family.[3]

Local public health authorities had responsibility for following up, visiting homes, inspecting latrines, jawboning people who lacked latrines to build them and people who had them to maintain these facilities well enough that members of the household would be willing to use them.

The two teams working in Jamaica needed slightly more than ten years to make their way across the island. When they began, under Washburn's predecessor in 1919, Jamaican children and many adults as well typically used the bush for defecation; even hospitals did not have satisfactory latrines; and most households had neither a latrine nor even a cesspit. Even in Kingston most people lacked access to any safe way to dispose of fecal matter. By the mid-1930s the schools were outfitted with separate latrines for boys and girls and sometimes with facilities for washing hands after toileting, most houses had a satisfactory latrine, and people in general used their latrines. Also important, Jamaicans demanded local public health services, even to the point of cooperating with the new corps of sanitary inspectors who visited their homes and businesses and, where needed, ordered improvements in sanitary facilities. In 1915 few Jamaicans associated defecation habits or excrement with disease; by 1930 most knew about the association in the case of hookworm, even though they may not have fully understood germ theory in relation to human waste. Washburn and his associates had used hookworms, a visible and repulsive sign of disease with obvious effects in the loss of energy and anemia, as a way to teach about disease transmission and methods of protecting against fecal disease.

When Jamaican school inspectors, asked specifically to comment on latrine access and use, reported around 1920, they wrote that few schools had latrines and, in those, although the children knew how to recite the lessons they had learned about why they should use latrines, they did not yet know how to use them and typically did not. Jamaican students lacked books, and the schools had almost no equipment. Students learned their lessons by rote, reciting what they heard their teachers say. By 1925 the inspectors found that most schools had latrines and students could both recite and practice latrine use. In the interim teachers had showed students how to use the school latrines, persuaded them to do so, and urged them to carry these lessons home to their parents. But the schools still lacked running water, so that children used the latrines without necessarily washing their hands afterwards or before eating lunch.[4]

As noted, in many countries it was agents from the Rockefeller Foundation who added the idea of reducing hookworm loads to local public health efforts. Initially, these agents sought to treat and cure hookworm directly, but often turned to education as their primary tool. In Jamaica, as we have seen, Ben Washburn found ways to reach schoolteachers and primary school students and to use the children to persuade their parents. In Mexico, by contrast, the Foundation achieved much less than did local initiatives begun under Secretary of Education José Vasconcelos in the early 1920s, continued by the *misioneros* in the later 1920s and by mostly female primary schoolteachers in the 1930s. And in Costa Rica efforts toward hookworm control began before Rockefeller Foundation agents appeared.

Meanwhile, Sri Lanka and Russia controlled cholera before they began to reduce mortality from other fecal disease, and in Sri Lanka cholera and some other types of fecal disease were brought under control in the general population more successfully than among plantation laborers. The Rockefeller agent in Sri Lanka, William Jacocks, found that the latrine people were most willing to use was one close to the front door of their house that was designed for household rather than shared village or neighborhood use.[5] Villagers were willing to take out a loan to buy the most expensive part of the latrine, the squatting plate, a metal or concrete slab with foot marks that covered the latrine pit. By 1930 the preferred pit was 20 feet deep and 5 feet in diameter, dug with a borer; a recycled metal barrel in the bottom assured that the pit would not cave in. Such a latrine would serve a single family for many years before becoming filled so that a new one had to be built. A Rockefeller official visiting Ceylon in 1915 found practically no latrines; visiting again in 1931, he found coverage ranging from 30 to 90 percent of households.[6] In Russia, where the Rockefeller Foundation did not operate, Soviet authorities urged cities to build or expand piped water and sewage systems, beginning in 1921. But in Leningrad the new sewage network was built of wood so that it soon deteriorated; by about 1930 the city's drinking water was again polluted.

As we have seen, sanitation improvements were generally more effective in the cities than in rural areas, and in the Americas this was sometimes assisted by the influence of the United States. In Panama, for example, Colon, Panama City, and the portions of the Canal Zone closest to the canal benefited more than the interior,[7] while in Cuba the programs of U.S. health authorities introduced in 1899 and their Cuban successors initially focused on Havana.

Japan controlled cholera, but typhoid fever remained a significant cause of death until around 1950. However, morbidity and mortality from other fecal disease were probably lower than elsewhere because of the long-standing Japanese practice of drinking tea made with boiled water and perhaps also because of the habit of bathing.

Most of the case-study countries, including Venezuela and Mexico, expanded access to health services for mothers, infants, and children in ways that may also have protected against fecal disease. But the key element in reducing exposure to fecal disease lay in informing people about the role of fecal matter in disease transmission and teaching them how to avoid exposure to feces. In many countries, including Japan, Korea, Costa Rica, and Jamaica in the period 1920–50 and in China in the 1950s, hygiene lessons in the schools taught primary-school-age students about fecal disease and how to avoid it. In those countries and elsewhere health authorities directed their efforts at adults as well, devising pictographs to illustrate the principles of disease transmission, the role of houseflies, the need to build latrines, and the construction of a latrine itself.

Mortality from some fecal disease declined in the period 1920–50 in at least nine of the case-study countries, as table 14 shows. The simultaneous beginning of persistent decline in infant mortality in most of these lands suggests that infants especially benefited from the control of fecal disease.

Malaria

The strategy of choice against malaria in the second half of the nineteenth century combined quinine treatments for individuals, usually without hospitalization, with attempts to drain swamps and marshes.[8] Both were old devices. In Europe (where a milder strain of malaria, *Plasmodium vivax,* prevailed) cinchona bark from South America, which contained quinine, was first used to treat fevers in the 1630s. By the mid-nineteenth century the Dutch were cultivating cinchona trees for quinine in Java, which expanded supply and reduced cost. Europeans had long deployed swamp drainage against the "bad air" for which malaria was named, and drainage projects are usually given some credit for the retreat of malaria in parts of Europe before 1900. But drainage systems tended to deteriorate, and because of their cost few locales were able to mount projects or fully to maintain what they did build.

Moreover, malaria had receded as a cause of death in many territories where little or nothing was attempted in the way of drainage. Leonard Jan Bruce-Chwatt and Julian de Zulueta argue that better housing, land reclamation, better agricultural practices, economic growth and a consequent higher standard of living, and sanitation all contributed to the early retreat of malaria in much of northwestern Europe, even though none of those things was undertaken with the specific intention of controlling the disease. Erwin H. Ackerknecht makes a similar case for the Upper Mississippi Valley of North America, adding some specifics.[9] Housing was better because it was more often screened to prevent access by insects, although not specifically mosquitoes. Agricultural techniques were better because farmers kept more livestock, which mosquitoes generally preferred to humans as sources of a meal. The declining price of quinine led to wider distribution while improvements in processing cinchona tree bark into a medicament, which began at the middle of the nineteenth century, standardized the drug's quality. Margaret Humphreys adds the interesting but still mostly untested idea that people in the American Midwest moved out of malaria areas, abandoning them.[10]

Although drainage and quinine dosing continued to be deployed, scientific advances in understanding the cycle of malaria began with Alphonse Laveran's 1880 identification of the malaria parasite and Ronald Ross's 1898 finding that culex mosquitoes play a central role in the transmission of malaria to birds. Giovanni Battista Grassi's identification in 1898 of anopheles mosquitoes as the vectors in human transmission clarified the task: combat malaria by locating the breeding and feeding sites of the strains of anopheles mosquitoes that played this role. From that point forward it was clear why swamps and marshes should be drained, but it also became evident that many other anti-mosquito activities might be useful.

Ross quickly decided that mosquito control would be more effective than treating victims with quinine. This implied a new approach: survey a locale to assess the scale of malaria and the location of people with the disease, discover which anopheles carried the disease, and locate their breeding and feeding sites. But he found it difficult to persuade important figures in public health or government to invest heavily enough to bring his ideas to success. Attempts at mosquito control led by Ross and others in Sierra Leone, Nigeria, India, Malaya, and Mauritius in the first decade of the new century had limited success at first. The techniques used, which attacked breeding sites, were effective enough, but they had to be repeated often. And, even when campaigns were limited to cities, the number of breeding sites was often too vast. Ross used thirty to forty men to fight mosquitoes in Freetown, Sierra Leone, but could never get the job done.[11] The same problem defeated this approach in Italy, where Angelo Celli concluded around 1900 that there were simply too many breeding sites, and in the Soviet Union, where one estimate indicated there were 38 million hectares of swamps and marshes in European Russia alone.[12] Moreover, some anopheles strains serving as vectors preferred to breed in puddles and small pools or in the still water at the edge of a river or stream, rather than swamps and marshes, making it yet more difficult to identify and eliminate all their breeding sites.

Thus up to the 1920s most governments trying to control malaria preferred to treat victims with quinine, which they might elect to subsidize or make available at no cost, as Italy did. At that point, however, even leading authorities remained uncertain about the optimal quinine dosage, many preferring a heavy dose once a week repeated for three or four months. By 1921 Ross preferred a dose of 10 grains, about 600 mg, a day for three or four months, which he expected to produce a cure.[13]

Quinine suppresses malarial fever so long as the parasites have not developed a resistance to this drug. Laveran observed that it also destroys the parasites while they feed inside red blood cells, and for a time in the 1890s leading authorities believed that quinine would kill all the parasites in a victim's blood. Celli found, however, that quinine did not kill gametocytes, the sexual form of the parasite, and that even people who had completed a course of quinine and who appeared to have recovered from malaria could still transmit the parasite to mosquitoes. Thus quinine relieves symptoms and allows people with malarial fevers to go back to work, but it is not a cure. Since it reduces the quantity of plasmodium in the bloodstream, the likelihood that malaria will be transmitted from one person to another drops. But it did not, and does not, provide a way to eradicate malaria.

As we have seen in chapter 5, a modified approach to malaria control was explored in Havana during the U.S. occupation of Cuba that began in 1898, and again in Panama from 1904 onward. This approach combined drainage, brush clearance, and filling in puddles and pools with additional measures designed to control the vector population, thereby reducing the opportunity for malaria to be transmitted from one person to another. Among this expanded array of measures some, including brush clearance, filling in puddles, and regrading road surfaces, were meant to destroy breeding sites, while others, including oiling (which prevented larvae from breathing) and the introduction of larvae-eating fish, were meant to prevent the development of adult mosquitoes, and still others, such as the use of screens and nets, would impede mosquito access to humans.[14]

Modifying the strategy of malaria control was not a simple or inexpensive step to take, however. Quinine could be distributed through the existing medical structure, using hospitals, clinics, and physicians in public and private practice. In addition, existing public institutions, such as post offices and police stations, were also used to distribute quinine directly to people with malaria, who learned when to dose themselves and how much to take. But steps to control the mosquito population or to impede access by the vectors to people would require an entirely different apparatus, which meant mobilizing resources for drainage projects or training and hiring people (such as Ross's mosquito brigades) to perform other steps toward insect control. An apparatus of either type had to be created in every country. Ross started in Freetown with a single man oiling puddles and pools, but soon understood that large teams—the mosquito brigades—would be required to oil, clear brush, sweep, fill, and channel. Moreover, some of the mosquito control steps performed by Ross in Sierra Leone and by William C. Gorgas in Cuba and Panama required cooperation from the local population, which first had to be educated about the role of mosquitoes in malaria transmission.

Among the countries considered in this study, where malaria was more often caused by the deadlier strain of the parasite *Plasmodium falciparum,* mortality declined not just in Cuba and Panama, under intensive campaigns led by U.S. authorities, but also from the 1920s or 1930s in Costa Rica, Jamaica, Mexico, and Venezuela (see table 14). Mortality may also have been retreating in Sri Lanka from the 1930s, although it certainly diminished at a faster pace during the DDT campaign begun in November 1945 than it had earlier. In the Soviet Union, where malaria was a major cause of death, mortality may have begun to recede in the period 1936–41.[15] But mortality from malaria did not begin to diminish in Albania, China, or the oil-rich countries of the Middle East until the late 1940s or thereafter. Thus the key concern here is to understand the techniques of malaria control that were used effectively in some countries before the introduction of DDT.

As noted, the intensive campaigns in Cuba and Panama followed the involvement of the United States in these countries. In Cuba U.S. authorities set out to control mosquitoes using a combination of oiling and inspections. In Panama they added larvae-eating fish, fines for failure to comply with regulations, brush clearance, and drainage, along with daily prophylactic doses of quinine. Elements of the Panama program involving discipline and fines could not readily be practiced outside military zones, and larvae-eating fish could be introduced only in bodies of water large enough to support them. Thus oiling played a key role. Inspection teams identified anopheles breeding sites, and oiled them often enough, usually weekly, to suppress mosquito populations.

These steps were actually an adaptation of control methods worked out first in British Malaya in 1900 and thereafter, and described by Malcolm Watson. One characteristic of this approach lies in its combination of surveys of breeding sites with drainage, clearance, and filling, oiling, screens, and quinine. Perhaps equally important, the mode of attack was modified for each area to accommodate problems specific to that locale.[16]

These labor-intensive methods required ongoing expenditures and work. During the 1920s this approach was substantially simplified by the introduction of a chemical larvicide, Paris green (copper acetoarsenate, a compound of copper and arsenic), which was cheaper and easier to work with than oil.[17] Dusting a breeding site with Paris green poisoned anopheles larvae when they broke the surface to feed. The main shortcoming of this larvicide recognized at the time was that it had to be reapplied once a month or even more often, requiring large numbers of people, boats, and dusting devices. (Since then Paris green has been shown to be widely toxic and to contribute to arsenic build-up in the environment.)

Paris green applications became the central method of mosquito control in Jamaica, Mexico, and Venezuela, while quinine doses continued for people already infected. In Jamaica public health authorities dusted rural areas; in urban areas, they identified sites where anopheles might breed and either dusted or tried to persuade homeowners to clean up those sites. Paris green was also used successfully in other countries, including Egypt, the American South, Puerto Rico, Transjordan, and the areas of Italy where the Rockefeller Foundation worked.[18]

But Paris green was not an effective method of mosquito control everywhere. Soviet authorities, learning of successful use of this cheap compound in the United States and Italy, experimented with it in the 1920s and 1930s, using aerial dusting. But they were not able to dust a wide enough area to have much impact on the incidence of malaria.[19]

The new home insecticide pyrethrum, derived from certain chrysanthemum varieties, had been introduced around 1911. Although it was not used extensively until around 1927, it may also have helped in towns and cities, especially in higher income households that could afford this product and in places where mosquito populations were comparatively light. It was used widely in Europe and the southern United States in the 1930s to kill mosquitoes on contact. And it was used successfully in worker barracks at South African estates.[20] Since it had no residual effect, however, repeated spraying was necessary. Humphreys argues that working class families in the American South probably could not afford to use it,[21] and this spray is rarely mentioned in sources on malaria control in low-income countries.

The use of oiling and Paris green and sometimes the insecticide pyrethrum, often combined with screening, inspections, and mosquito brigades, suggested a new orientation for mosquito control, which directed efforts not at swamps or marshes, or at entire regions, but at each site where malaria vectors bred and each locale where people had malaria. Many authorities argued that what the United States had done in Panama was simply too costly to be repeated elsewhere. But malaria control campaigns in Jamaica, Mexico, and Venezuela all showed that low-income countries could mobilize enough of these local measures against mosquitoes to control the disease and to reduce mortality quite substantially.[22] It seems clear that no one approach would have worked everywhere.[23] But it also seems to be the case that the local-design approach would have had a wider effect if it had been attempted in more places.

Once it became available, DDT proved more efficacious because of its residual effects. It could be sprayed on walls inside the house, and in that form would continue to kill mosquitoes for a lengthy period. Or, mixed with oil, it could be used as a larvicide, though in that form DDT has to be reapplied about as often as Paris green had been. DDT produced faster mosquito control and more abrupt declines in malaria mortality in the period 1945–55, but ultimately at the cost of much more severe toxic effects in the environment than oiling, Paris green, or pyrethrum. (It is worth noting that at about the same time synthetic forms of quinine also contributed to malaria control.)[24]

Malaria rebounded in many countries as DDT was withdrawn from use, but mortality did not rise as much as morbidity. For the early twenty-first century, estimates of new cases each year range from 500 million to much higher numbers, and deaths from 1 to 3 million.[25]

Tuberculosis

In the late nineteenth century pulmonary tuberculosis, then usually called consumption or phthisis, was the leading cause of death in several Western countries. Urbanization, which meant that more people lived in crowded dwellings, and industrialization, which meant that more people worked in crowded factories, had proved to be allies of the disease. Mortality from tuberculosis began to decline in some countries between the 1870s and the 1890s, however. Although there is not yet universal agreement about how to explain this decline, the leading hypothesis is that rising numbers of people with active cases were being isolated, with the secondary hypothesis that nutrition improved and specifically that protein intake rose.[26] In fact, relatively small numbers of people with pulmonary tuberculosis were removed from their homes and workplaces to be treated in clinics, hospitals, and sanatoriums that specialized in tuberculosis cases, and the annual pace of retreat in tuberculosis mortality was slow. (In Western Europe tuberculosis mortality declined at an annual rate of some one to two percent from the late nineteenth century to the 1940s, despite a number of changes in treatment regimens. The pace quickened only when antibiotics were introduced.) The treatments given in sanatoriums, which stressed a generous diet with milk and eggs, as well as prolonged rest followed by limited exercise, probably had some good effect, slowing the development of the disease. But it appears to have been isolation that made the difference.[27] Many patients recovered well enough to resume their everyday lives, although there was no cure. What treatment offered was a good prospect of transforming an active case back into an inactive infection and, with the home regimen that sanatorium doctors and nurses taught their patients, a chance to prevent reinfection or reactivation.

Treatment in a specialized facility was always expensive. Even in the richest countries of the period, such as Britain and the United States, working people and the poor could not afford to pay for such facilities, because of both cost and wages foregone. Their isolation in sanatoriums depended on subsidies from private charity or other sources, rather than fees paid by the sick. Beginning around 1900 anti-tuberculosis associations organized campaigns in many Western countries to raise money, some of which went to provide charity beds in sanatoriums.

Robert Koch's 1882 discovery of the bacteria associated with tuberculosis did not bring a quick change in ideas about how to treat or to prevent tuberculosis, but it did draw attention to sputum, where live bacteria were found in samples taken from people with active cases of the disease. (Thus the disappearance of live bacteria in sputum was a sign that an active case had retreated to the status of an infection.) By about 1900 health authorities in many Western countries had organized campaigns against spitting on grounds that the spit of tuberculosis victims contained bacteria, which might infect other people. Later research showed that the bacteria, seated in the lungs, are brought into the mouth in sputum (the mucus brought up from the lungs), and more often disseminated through coughing and sneezing, which blast droplets of moisture containing bacteria into the air around the person with an active case, than through spitting, which directs the bacteria-laden moisture toward the ground. Healthy people may breathe in the droplets, giving bacteria access to their lungs and the opportunity to initiate an infection. Those already infected may be reinfected by this route and convert to an active case. Thus, living or working with someone with an active case vastly increases the likelihood of becoming infected or of developing an active case through reinfection. Skin tests, introduced in 1907 and 1908, showed that in fact many people in Western countries had been infected, though only some of them had developed active cases.[28]

As noted, most low-income countries could not afford the isolation approach to tuberculosis treatment and prevention, although the Soviet Union managed to add substantially to the number of sanatoriums in the decade 1927–37.[29] Sanatoriums and other facilities were too expensive to build, staff, and maintain on the scale required to turn mortality downward; the overwhelming majority of patients could not afford to pay for sanatorium treatment; and attempts to raise money to build sanatoriums and pay for treatment for the poor developed more slowly than in richer lands or failed altogether.[30] Low-income countries also could rarely afford lung-collapse therapy, the briefly popular the surgical intervention that Western countries adopted in the 1930s, or the improved diagnostic X-rays used more often in the 1930s and 1940s. Thus, leading elements of the Western approach to tuberculosis diagnosis and treatment were unavailable, or only selectively available, outside the West.

Because sanatorium treatment was expensive, physicians devised rules of behavior to aid in recovery at home. They hoped these regimens would further assist recovery and the ongoing battle against reactivation of the disease. Beginning around 1900 people with active cases, those inside sanatoriums and those still living at home as well, were urged to spit into pocket spittoons or to catch their spit and the product of their sneezing in handkerchiefs, which would then be disinfected, such as by boiling them. By the 1910s many of the national organizations formed in Western countries to combat tuberculosis were also hiring home visitors to help identify people with tuberculosis, advise them about treatment, and educate them in the need to control their sputum in order to protect people in the household from infection or re-infection.

These inexpensive methods of tuberculosis management could be adopted in low-income countries. They do not seem to have been used extensively in Japan, where mortality remained high until after World War II.[31] In Moscow dispensaries and sanatoria were never numerous enough to serve everyone with tuberculosis, but Michael David finds that health education reached large numbers of people in that city, where official data indicate that mortality was declining, although he does not attempt to account for the pattern of decline.[32] But in several countries studied here, including Costa Rica, Panama, Cuba, Jamaica, and Venezuela (as noted in table 14), tuberculosis mortality declined between the 1920s and the late 1940s, that is, in the period before antibiotic treatment began to become available. Mortality from this disease also declined in some other countries in the same period, including Argentina and Uruguay.[33] Only one of these cases, Jamaica, has been studied in enough detail to suggest how that decline was achieved.

Jamaica's physicians, as we have seen, were mostly British, who worked as civil servants in this and other colonies. They kept themselves well enough informed about treatment ideas in Britain to be able to recommend those in Jamaica, so that the idea of sequestering patients in clinics, tuberculosis wings of hospitals, and sanatoriums was in circulation in Jamaica by the 1910s. But the Home Office insisted that each colony be self-supporting, and Jamaica did not generate enough revenue to pay for such facilities. Although some people were treated in tuberculosis wings of hospitals beginning in 1927, it was not until 1940 that the first sanatorium was opened. In the meantime, tuberculosis mortality had declined sharply. Even though tuberculin testing showed that the proportion of people surveyed who had been exposed to tuberculosis was increasing, fewer people were developing active cases. Afro-Jamaicans, however, still developed active cases more frequently than did blacks or whites in the United States, and among Afro-Jamaicans the disease progressed more rapidly.

Since isolation of the sick in institutions was not yet a practical option, health educators and home visitors in Jamaica began in the 1910s to concentrate on things that people could do for themselves. A. Bruce McFarlane extracted simple lessons from germ theory and disseminated those through schoolteachers and primary school students in a pamphlet published in 1912. McFarlane and other health educators explained how to recognize tuberculosis, why the well should try to avoid contact with the sick, and why it was necessary to get people with the disease to sneeze and spit into handkerchiefs that would be burned, boiled, disinfected, or buried. In a broad public health campaign begun in 1926, Jamaicans were encouraged to disinfect or bury the sputum of people with the disease and to provide the sick a separate room for sleeping or, if that could not be done, to build a separate hut outside the house for them. In any event children in the household of a sick person were to be sent to live with relatives or friends. During the 1930s public health nurses supervised cases at home. By 1940, when the first sanatorium opened and nearly a decade before the introduction of effective drugs, tuberculosis mortality in Jamaica had diminished to a level similar to that in the United States and in northern Europe.[34]

If the European model of tuberculosis control will not explain the retreat of this disease in many countries between the 1920s and the 1940s, Jamaican practice, adapted from advice developed by European and American physicians, offers an alternative explanation. There are some signs that its main elements—learning how to identify tuberculosis, changing some behaviors in people with the disease, and sequestering the sick at home—were used elsewhere. Advice about home treatment began to appear in Western countries in 1889 in the form of brief pamphlets written for popular use. In 1910 Hyslop Thomson, the medical superintendent of the Liverpool sanatorium, opened his guide for patients with this observation: "in the warfare against consumption the influence of education occupies a foremost place." The patient with tuberculosis needed to have "an intimate knowledge" of the causes of this disease; specifically, patients and the general public needed to know that home conditions played a much larger role in spread of tuberculosis than did inheritance from a parent.[35] Thus healthy individuals assumed responsibility for keeping themselves well, and tuberculosis patients, for avoiding the infection of others. One pamphlet, Adolphus Knopf's 1899 *Tuberculosis as a Disease of the Masses and How to Combat It,* enjoyed an unusually wide circulation in the United States and was also translated into twenty-seven languages.[36] Knopf's later books on the same topic, in 1901 *Tuberculosis as a Disease of the Masses* and in 1909 *Tuberculosis: A Preventable and Durable Disease,* also went into many editions and were translated into other languages. Knopf emphasized home treatment, the safe disposal of sputum, and how to avoid droplet infection, and he argued that people who were not infected did not need to worry about infection even from a family member if they took appropriate steps.[37]

Home treatment is an aspect of prevention and management that has not yet received much attention from scholars, who have concentrated their researches on the sanatorium movement and on discrimination against people with tuberculosis.[38] Its apparent success in Jamaica raises the possibility that home treatment played a significant role in the decline of tuberculosis mortality in Western countries and elsewhere in the period 1900–1950.[39] In Jamaica slightly less crowded housing and better nutrition may also have contributed, but it is unlikely that protein intake increased. The leading explanation for the retreat of tuberculosis there lies in changes in individual behavior that protected people who had not yet been infected or who had not yet developed active cases. Such changes remained a leading part of the advice physicians and nurses in the United States and Britain gave to tuberculosis patients and their family members into the 1940s, up to the point when antibiotics became available.[40] In the Soviet Union home treatment was still, of necessity, the leading treatment in the years after World War II.[41]

Conclusion

Control of fecal disease, malaria, and tuberculosis was uneven. Some countries made substantial progress, some made limited progress, some made no progress, and some regressed in the period 1920–50.

For fecal disease the most important technology was the pit latrine, and the most important intervention was people learning why they needed to build and maintain latrines. Properly built and situated, latrines protected people from fecal contamination of water used for drinking and food preparation.

The techniques of malaria control that worked so well in Jamaica, Mexico, and Venezuela either did not work as well in some other countries, such as the Soviet Union, or were not tried. The introduction of DDT led to faster progress, and its effectiveness persuaded countries where earlier malaria-control techniques had not been tried, or had been tried without conviction, to use DDT. There are thus two obvious differences between the effects achieved by DDT and those achieved by the techniques in use between about 1920 and 1943: the pace of control was faster with DDT, and DDT was used more widely.

The same thing is true with streptomycin and the drugs later developed for use against tuberculosis. The pace of tuberculosis control was faster with the new biomedicines and, because they quickly became available at low prices, they were used more widely than the techniques of isolation of the sick and education of both the sick and the well, which had formed the centerpiece of efforts against tuberculosis in earlier decades. These new medicines quickened the pace of control even in the countries where tuberculosis had been declining as a cause of death for many decades, such as England and Wales. Wherever they were used, the new drugs allowed the control of tuberculosis to move toward the hopeful point of the early 1970s, when many informed observers hoped for the global eradication of pulmonary tuberculosis. Since the 1980s tuberculosis has been recognized as resurgent, often in association with drug resistance. In the face of resistance even to second- and third-line drug combination therapies, it may be useful to reexamine the successful methods of tuberculosis control employed before the biomedicines were introduced.

Despite the unevenness of progress among the twelve case-study countries in controlling fecal disease, malaria, and tuberculosis in the 1920s and 1930s, what is most important to notice is that so many countries managed to reduce mortality from these diseases before the appearance of DDT and antibiotics. They relied largely on things people could do for themselves. On this score there is a striking similarity between the public health programs implemented in the Soviet Union, where "the protection of the health of the workers is the task of the workers themselves,"[42] and those followed in Jamaica, Cuba, Costa Rica, and elsewhere, where health authorities offered direction and advice, but ordinary people had to learn and do the things necessary for disease control. Low-income countries found low-cost ways to control these diseases, relying more heavily on educating people to do things for themselves and less on public financing, expert intervention, medical technology, or hospitals and other health care facilities.

Making individuals aware of health risks and how to cope with them has come to be widely recognized as an essential feature of reducing mortality from lung cancer, heart disease, and other maladies associated with diet and lifestyle. What this chapter shows is that fecal disease and tuberculosis, and to a lesser degree malaria, were all combated by a similar mode, which informed ordinary people in accessible terms about how these diseases operated and how people could protect themselves from them. Those things—self-awareness and self-help—were the central feature of disease protection in the low-income countries in the early decades of their health transitions.

Conclusion

What do we learn from this study of countries that achieved high levels of longevity without high levels of income?

Except for Oman and perhaps some of the other oil-rich countries of the Middle East and North Africa, the countries considered in this study began their health transitions between the 1890s and the 1920s or 1930s. At the point of initiation they resembled one another in having high mortality, although the levels varied among them, and in confronting fecal disease, malaria, and tuberculosis as leading causes of death. Many of these countries made rapid gains in survival in the 1920s, 1930s, and into the 1940s, that is, before the introduction of antibiotics and DDT and before vaccines other than for smallpox were widely used. Although in the 1950s none of them quite matched the high-survival countries of that day in life expectancy at birth, they had by then claimed an exceptional position, which distinguished them as countries with much higher survival than could be expected from the level of income.

Once they had achieved that level of survival, however, their paths diverged. Japan went on in the years from 1947 into the 1970s to become a global leader in both life expectancy and GDPpc, transforming itself so decisively that few recalled its prior status as a country with good health but low income. South Korea followed, adding to survival at a rapid pace in the twenty years after 1953 and then, during the 1960s, beginning to move toward its late-century position as a middle-income country. Its earlier status as a low-income country with good health, too, was lost from sight.

Mexico may actually have begun its health transition earlier than any other country considered, even as early as the 1860s, but it did not make either steady or substantial progress until the 1920s and 1930s. After having established itself as a low-income country with high life expectancy, Mexico grew slowly into its position as a middle-income country. Venezuela began to make progress in survival later than Mexico, in the 1920s or 1930s. By the 1950s life expectancy surpassed what could be expected from its level of income. Venezuela, too, then went on to join the ranks of the middle-income countries.

Russia, Ukraine, China, and Albania began health transitions within the period from the 1890s to the 1930s, Russia probably first among them. They made exceptionally rapid gains in survival from the late 1940s into the 1960s, so that by 1960 all of them stood out for having levels of life expectancy higher than could be projected from their income levels. After that, however, all of them faltered in both income and life expectancy; Albania alone managed to resume survival gains, at least according to official estimates. Russia and China dismantled the health and social systems they had built, respectively, in the 1920s and 1930s and in the 1950s and 1960s, and in that disassembly saw survival stop improving or, in Russia, actually regress.

Sri Lanka, Costa Rica, Panama, Cuba, and Jamaica all began to add years of survival between the 1890s and the 1920s, and all managed to make rapid progress from the 1920s onward. By the 1950s all five stood out as countries with good health but low income. According to the expectations of some theorists, the social growth they had managed to achieve by the 1950s should have promoted them into sustained economic growth. Costa Rica managed to break into the ranks of the middle-income countries but Sri Lanka, Cuba, and Jamaica remained low-income lands. These are the archetypal cases whose success in health is the most impressive, because it began and remained so thoroughly detached from success at economic growth. Panama appears to fit this model as well, but its health achievement may be an effect of averaging well-reported high survival in the Canal Zone area with poorly reported low survival elsewhere.

In all of these countries progress in survival occurred despite ongoing signs of poor nutrition, and in some countries even amid periodic famines. Higher protein diets, food intake distributed across the year, and diets balanced in vitamins and minerals came decades after these countries had begun to make sustained additions to life expectancy.

Then there are the outliers, the oil-rich lands of the Middle East and North Africa, which successfully used their oil revenues to elevate the health statistics of their populations in an exceptionally short space of time. The most thoroughly documented case among these is Oman, which may have followed a lead taken by Kuwait. But all seven—Algeria and Libya in North Africa, and Iran, Iraq, Kuwait, Oman, and Saudi Arabia in the Middle East—invested much more heavily and directly in social growth than any other countries examined in this study, quickly building up both the facilities and the personnel required for modern establishments in education and medicine and, in the cities, public health as well. But for oil, all of them were low-income countries. They managed to use oil and autocratic decisions about how petroleum revenues would be spent to fund a hothouse scheme of rapid social development to improve survival and well-being in their populations.

In this study the group of countries examined has deliberately been enlarged and made more diverse than the traditionally cited examples of Sri Lanka and Costa Rica, which are always used as instances of low-income countries with good health. This larger group underscores one of the principal findings of modern research into how life expectancy gains have been achieved, which is that different countries have found their own paths to gains in life expectancy. Despite the countries' resemblances at the outset, no two stories are identical, nor even particularly similar. What stands out among these case studies, diverse as they are, however, is the adoption of strategies of social growth and common ideas about disease control and avoidance. Even in the oil-rich lands, which had the widest range of opportunities for adopting new policies, the decision made was to invest in social development, and that decision paid off not just in social growth but also in rapid life expectancy gains. In Venezuela larger investments in economic growth returned smaller rewards, assessed by how far they matched expectations, than did smaller but persistent investments in public health, education, and health care. In the oil-rich lands of Asia and North Africa autocratic decisions led to the creation of the instruments of public health, education, and health care that allowed rapid and substantial gains in life expectancy.

In important ways social growth that did not lead a country to high-income status may in the long run prove to be a more useful mode of development for other low-income countries. It is markedly less abusive in its exploitation of scarce resources, and it avoids the agonies associated with the early stages of industrial modernization. The low-income countries' model of social growth also sets a different goal. Whereas economic growth measures success by adding to income, improving material life, and meeting people's expectations for a continually rising standard of living, social growth sets the goal of self- and community improvement. It concentrates results on what is absolutely the fundamental prize, which is good health and survival. A global strategy of social growth would also produce less inequality among nations in income and wealth, hence lead to a more ethically defensible and morally acceptable distribution of material goods. And it would make middle-income rather than high-income status the goal. Imagine a world in which the most valued skills and ideas lead not to the possession of ever more consumer goods but to improvement of the quality of life for individuals and the community.

In the Western model of social development, worked out in Europe beginning in the 1880s and explained by Peter Lindert, economic development led to and allowed social growth. There open and democratic political regimes, at the beginning mostly in Protestant countries, drew from their economic wealth to invest in education, public health, and health care—hospitals and dispensaries, the training of nurses and doctors, pensions, and health insurance—and eventually to build welfare states. A different style of social development emerged in the low-income countries studied here. Protestantism played a negligible role among these countries, of which only Jamaica was mostly Protestant. Nor did having open and democratic political regimes contribute. Venezuela and Mexico excepted, the countries examined here were either colonies, in which decisions were made partly in the metropole and partly among elites in the colony, or authoritarian regimes. Some of the colonies, such as Jamaica and Sri Lanka, were governed by stable regimes, but political instability was often characteristic of these countries.

Among the lands in this study, in fact, colonization appears often as a positive factor. Britain both allowed and encouraged social growth in Sri Lanka and Jamaica before those two countries gained local autonomy, in 1931 and 1944 respectively, and in the years leading up to independence as well. Imperial Japan introduced improvements in public health and education in Korea and Taiwan, as did the United States in Cuba, the Canal Zone portion of Panama, and Puerto Rico. But of course many other countries under colonial control failed to improve survival, and Britain, Japan, the United States, and other countries often pursued their own interests at the expense of their colonies.

Because the lands studied in this book were low-income countries when they began their social growth, they could afford much less than the wealthier countries of the West could even in the 1880s, when those countries began their own social development. The low-income countries per-

force focused on a smaller though not a uniform set of social improvements, in the five areas of social growth identified in the introduction:
primary schooling, inexpensive public health improvements, broader access to rudimentary health care, popular understanding of health risks and
how to avoid them, and the involvement of the people in public health
endeavors. It is noteworthy that only in a few cases did all five elements
of social growth emerge. Jamaicans lacked ready access to health care until the 1970s, though the other four elements began building there in the
1910s and 1920s. China deferred universal schooling and literacy until after having achieved a distinctive position as a low-income land with high
life expectancy, but the Patriotic Hygiene Campaign of the 1950s and the
Cooperative Medical System associated with the barefoot doctors did use
indoctrination and mass participation in common health goals to spread
basic information about health risks. None of the oil-rich lands of the Middle East and North Africa emphasized popular participation in public
health improvements, except quite indirectly, in the form of people moving into cities where such amenities could be supplied much more readily than they could be in rural areas or to nomadic peoples. Thus, we can
conclude that three or four of these five elements of social growth were
sufficient to transform survival prospects.

A second common factor is that, despite their low income levels, all
these lands possessed a certain degree of prior development. Maddison's
estimates of GDPpc capture one form of that prior development: all had
surpassed the threshold of per capita income equivalent to some 1990 I$
1,000. All had basic systems of transportation and communication that
reached into their interiors and linked them to other countries. Many had
small governments of limited means.

More important still is that all the countries considered here that initiated health transitions by the 1930s—that is, all but the oil-rich lands of
North Africa and the Middle East—had the capacity for social growth
despite the meager amounts available to invest in it. By about 1900 these
countries possessed the social organization necessary to emulate Sweden,
which had been able to institute a systematic program of vaccination
against smallpox a century before, though few did that quite as rapidly
or as effectively as Sweden had. Some of them managed also to use quarantines to control cholera. All of them had populations in which people
valued schools highly enough to help build rudimentary structures, find
teachers, and carry forward the process of primary schooling. All of them
had people who were willing to learn new things about how to protect
themselves from the health risks they faced, and to adopt new modes of

behavior. Even where social growth programs were paternalistic, as they were in Mexico, rural people cooperated in schooling, latrine-building, and other programs.

Like the Western nations, these countries clearly invested in education, public health, and health care. Most invested in primary schools and primary-school teachers without expecting those investments to pay off as much in better health as in better economic opportunities. But health education was usually emphasized, and some effects of this education came quickly, as happened in Jamaica, where children practiced new hygiene rules for using pit latrines and taught their parents those rules. More effects came after a lag, during which the children who learned health rules in school grew up to practice those rules in their own lives and as parents. The countries that invested in schools, schooling, and often also in health education appear to have laid a firmer foundation for ongoing social development and continuing gains in survival than did the countries that turned to regimentation to disseminate health lessons. It is striking to notice that Cuba and Jamaica were able to sustain progress in survival though lengthy periods of hard times in the latter decades of the twentieth century, while the Russian Federation, China, and Ukraine were not.

Most of these countries invested also in public health. They built some high-cost water and sewage facilities in the main cities, but could rarely expand those to provide services even to the entire urban population. In rural areas and in the poorer sections of their cities they turned instead to latrine building, education of the public in the fact of diseases being spread through fecal matter, and lessons on how to control those diseases. They inspected houses, businesses, and public buildings for compliance, and they often demanded that people follow the new rules, levying fines, as in Panama, or using the ideal of the new citizen in a state responsible for public health, as in the Soviet Union, Albania, and China. In the 1920s, 1930s, and into the 1940s public health improvements played the leading role in controlling disease and increasing survival. Even in the oil-rich lands, with their later start and emphasis on direct heath care, urbanization and the concentration of public health improvements in cities, especially improvements delivering safe water and removing human waste, acted as an important ally of survival gains in the period after about 1960.

All of these countries tried early on in their social development efforts to make health care more accessible, to train more doctors and sometimes also more nurses, often to train less skilled cadres of health providers, and to build more hospitals. Investments in physicians and hospitals contributed comparatively little to better survival, however, because beds and doctors were so costly to provide. Investments in more democratic access to health care and to health information paid better returns. Many countries, from Russia with its feldshers to Mexico with its rural schoolteachers acting as health aides, tried to give people an avenue to treatment and better information about health risks and how to avoid them. It was not until the 1950s and 1960s in oil-rich lands of the Middle East and North Africa that more medical providers with extensive training, more hospitals, and eventually better medical technology made a striking contribution to progress in survival. As of 2000, the costliest elements of medicine were still no more than selectively available in Cuba, Costa Rica, Jamaica, Panama, and Sri Lanka. Yet those countries matched the rich countries in life expectancy and even surpassed some of them.

Perhaps a more surprising finding is that despite the characteristics of the three lands upon which attention has usually been concentrated — Costa Rica, Kerala state, and Sri Lanka in the 1960s and afterwards — issues of social justice also did not play a significant role in social growth in the formative early stages, up to about 1950. Such factors as fair-price food shops and more equitable access to better housing or granting females more autonomy in education, family decisions, or community and national decision-making certainly made a difference in the 1960s and thereafter, but they are striking for their near absence in the earlier period. Jamaica managed to provide females with equality and then an advantage in schooling opportunities by 1900, but in most of the low-income lands considered here female schooling and literacy continued to lag male until much later. And in Jamaica educational opportunity for females has still not been translated into an equal place for women in business or political leadership positions.

In this account paternalism was a more important driving force than Protestantism, democracy, or popular demands for social development. Colonial and imperial authorities, communists who shared a vision of social progress developed by the intelligentsia rather than by the people, and autocrats and dictators in oil-rich lands made most of the decisions about where, when, and how much to invest in social growth. It is nevertheless important that the people bought into these plans, no doubt at least in part because social growth was intended to improve the well-being of ordinary people, turning in every case away from a past in which elites benefited most from public sector spending.

The European countries that began social development in the 1880s did not foresee that the steps they took would lead to the welfare state. The low-income countries studied here did not, in developing schools, public health practices, broader health care facilities, and informed and participatory populations, see themselves as specifically adopting policies of social growth. That term and the idea of a coherent program of social development in low-income countries did not appear until the 1950s and 1960s in efforts made by United Nations officials to conceptualize a type of development in which low-income countries might participate.

Practice thus preceded theory, in a disorganized way and from quite different sources of inspiration. The reasons Jamaicans prized schooling for their children in the 1910s and 1920s, which anticipated better jobs and higher status, and made the local efforts required to provide their children with schools and teachers, bear little resemblance to the ideas behind the democratization of schooling in the Soviet Union in the 1920s and 1930s and the emergence of the idea that the children of workers could be physicians, engineers, political leaders, or indeed anything they wished.

Although many people in the low-income lands that achieved high life expectancy shared the faith that Europeans were then developing in the power of education to improve the human condition, in the power of public health improvements and access to health care to reduce disease risks, and in the value of what people could learn and do for themselves, there is no evidence, nor even any hint, of coordination or cooperation among these countries in planning social growth. But there was a sense of shared confidence in European and U.S. models of schools, of public health rules, inspectors, and authorities; and of hygiene education, and an interest in adapting those models to local circumstances. In general the leaders of social innovations knew a great deal about European and U.S. models in education, public health, and medicine. And in general the wider public accepted those models.

In contrast, when in the 1950s some UN officials began to write about social development, they appear to have known little about what had already been achieved in some low-income lands.[1] Their interest in an alternative model of development to industrialization was certainly not acknowledged to have come from prior achievements in any of the countries considered here, or any other low-income lands, and it was not until the 1970s that scholars began to write seriously and in an informed way about some cases of social growth in low-income lands.

As theories of social growth began to emerge in the 1960s and 1970s, the United Nations remained a leading promoter of development.[2] Then and since, these theories have pointed in two directions: first, that social development will lead to economic development, and second, that social development will improve the quality of life and survival itself.

But this study suggests that there is another way to think about coordination and inspiration. In all of the countries studied here, large numbers of people died prematurely from malaria, tuberculosis, and fecal disease, but by the 1910s and 1920s, these diseases could be successfully combated. The methods of controlling them came to be understood partly through medical and public health research in Western countries and partly through what Western public health experts learned while working in Latin America, the Caribbean, and Asia. For malaria key discoveries occurred in the years surrounding 1900: certain mosquitoes with certain habits and habitats transmitted malaria, and those mosquitoes and their larvae could successfully be controlled by larvicides, larvae-eating fish, pesticides, and the destruction of breeding sites. For tuberculosis the key finding was that the disease was communicated through matter coughed or sneezed by someone with an active case. The sick could protect the well from infection by managing these things, especially by catching their discharges from mouth and nose. And the healthy could protect themselves by learning to recognize the symptoms of tuberculosis in someone else and by safeguarding themselves from exposure. And for fecal disease what mattered most was the basic association of human fecal matter with disease and disease transmission. Disposed of properly, such as in a pit latrine, fecal matter posed much less risk or none at all. The key step was to persuade people to build, maintain, and use latrines, and to wash their hands after toileting.

Each of these steps toward disease control depended on things people learned to do for themselves. None of the steps necessary to manage these diseases and exposure to them was costly, even for people with very low incomes. Each required much more in new information and behaviors than in new investments. Even the schools where hygiene lessons were taught were inexpensive structures, staffed by poorly paid teachers, possessing practically no equipment, even few books. (Among the most remarkable features in disease control is that a number of low-income lands succeeded in reducing mortality from tuberculosis earlier than did Japan, where successful control developed only after World War II.)

What is suggested by these histories of people learning how to protect themselves against disease is that there is already a historical laboratory available to be consulted in two circumstances that matter especially in the present day. First, the body of individual-level experience with disease control surveyed here shows how people in the past, often people with only a few years schooling, learned about communicable disease and its management. Those lessons remain available for countries that have not achieved the phase of social growth and for people who have never learned such things. Second, the techniques used to teach people about communicable diseases can, at least in many cases, also be applied to teach people throughout the world about how to cope with the diet and lifestyle threats associated with chronic diseases that are growing health problems for the present and the future. In other words, for chronic diseases, too, it is not necessary to rely just on high-cost medicine and surgery, and on the attempt to correct problems after they appear.

Even the use of lower-cost options such as antibiotics and DDT may not be as significant as is generally thought. Japan and the Soviet Union both introduced their own antibiotics during World War II, but most of the low-income countries did not have wide access to antibiotics until the late 1940s, at the earliest. Although little has so far been learned about the dissemination of these drugs outside the West, the opinion has become firmly entrenched in scholarly work that antibiotics accounted for a major improvement in survival across Africa, Asia, and Latin America as early as the 1940s and certainly in the 1950s and 1960s by reducing mortality from bacterial diseases. That interpretation is consistent with the observation that, in this period, it became generally possible for countries to initiate health transitions at lower levels of GDPpc, below I\$ 1,000, than had earlier been typical. DDT was deployed beginning in 1943 but more widely from 1947 to control anopheles mosquitoes and some other disease vectors. Antibiotics and DDT sharply expanded the power of the techniques of disease and vector control previously used. But these new chemicals did not necessarily prove to be lasting contributors to continued progress in survival. Whereas Sri Lanka, Costa Rica, Cuba, Jamaica, and Mexico managed to keep their health transitions going in the 1980s and 1990s, many of the low-income countries that began transitions in the 1940s saw those transitions weaken in the face of HIV/AIDS, resurgent malaria and tuberculosis, and the never-solved problems of widespread fecal disease. It proved easier to control tuberculosis in the 1920s and 1930s, before the introduction of antibiotics effective in its treatment, than to control HIV/AIDS in the 1980s and 1990s.

By controlling fecal disease, malaria, and tuberculosis before the introduction of DDT or antibiotics and vaccines appropriate to these diseases, these countries displayed a much greater capacity than is commonly recognized to manage disease without relying on advanced medical technology and modern medicines. The now rich lands for the most part did the same thing, controlling fecal disease and tuberculosis, and some of them, including the United States, also malaria before introduction of the biochemical means for doing that. Today it may often be faster to use biomedicine to control bacterial diseases, but this is not the only way and it may not be the best way. Taking this approach may forgo the step in which individual people learn how diseases are transmitted and what they can do to impede transmission and protect themselves against disease. This approach may also lead us toward exaggerated confidence in medicines and chemistry and too much reliance on them. We may wait to try vigorous management of new diseases, such as HIV/AIDS, until we have appropriate antiviral medicines and vaccines. Worse, we may lose confidence in people's capacity to take care of themselves, once they are armed with the information they need about disease risks and how to control those risks.

The high-income countries have a huge advantage in high-cost medicine. They have created this medicine and found ways to deploy it widely, although seldom universally, in their own populations. They have not, however, found ways to deploy high-cost medicine in middle- and low-income countries. Some important steps have been taken, not least among them the eradication of smallpox, the approaching eradication of polio, the immunization of children in many poor countries against commonplace diseases, and, most recently, the promise to make HIV/AIDS drugs widely available. Even so, such efforts are little more than a drop in the bucket. Pick any low-income country and look up recent surveys of its inventory of the equipment and personnel of high-cost medicine, including even some of the older and less expensive items such as kidney dialysis and X-ray machines. The story is always the same: these countries lack the equipment and the personnel necessary to make modern medicine available on terms approaching those of the high-income countries. Even after decades of availability, this technology remains selectively accessible to sick people.

We cannot wait for economic development to transform low- and middle-income countries into rich lands. The historical record shows economic progress that is entirely too skimpy and fragmentary. And although the point is much less often made, we also cannot wait for medical innovations made in rich countries to make their way to poor lands. This process, too, is skimpy and fragmentary, and altogether inadequate to the task.

In the 1990s the World Bank began to engage more directly in population health, assessing health problems and extending loans to develop health and education resources in low and middle-income countries.[3] New players, including the Bill and Melinda Gates Foundation and the Global

Fund to Fight AIDS, Tuberculosis and Malaria, have more recently made funds available to buy medications to treat HIV/AIDS and for other purposes.[4] The future direction of such investments is at stake now. Should they be aimed chiefly at treating the sick and managing diseases already present, or toward preventing future cases of disease? Low- and high-income countries face contrasting risks to health, but they confront the same debate: which will do the most to improve population health, medicine or public health, with its emphasis on disease prevention?

The rapid rise of life expectancy in the oil-rich lands of the Middle East and North Africa shows what money can do. But today most of the world lacks anything approaching resources of that scale or any hope of attaining them in the near future. Today the world needs a plan for development that will serve countries where incomes and life expectancy are both unacceptably low. The information collected here and the interpretations made of it suggest that this plan should have three elements.

First, the country that may benefit from social growth in this model must already have a certain level of development. It is probably no longer useful to think rigidly about that 1990 I$ 1,000 as a threshold. What matters more as an index is whether a country and its people possess the capacity to organize and manage programs in such areas as primary schooling, health education, devising low-cost strategies to solve public health problems, and taking useful advantage of briefly trained medical aids.

The second element is to promote the goal of social development in some combination of education, public health, medicine, and popular participation that suits local preferences and serves local needs. The foundational ideas of social growth and disease control are already available, though they need to be tailored to today's challenges. Today it is still important in many lands to control fecal disease, malaria, and tuberculosis, but it is also important to control HIV/AIDS, diabetes, and coronary heart disease. Thus, while it is a good idea to treat people with HIV or AIDS with retroviral drugs, it is another good and necessary thing to engage people not yet sick in avoiding infection. The best solution to these diseases, and others, lies not in treatment of the sick, but in prevention.

This leads us to the final element. For some decades now medicine has had the upper hand in the minds of policy makers, in a manner analogous to the preference for economic over social development in the same group. Many students of human survival believe that public health and its potential contributions to disease prevention should be given more importance. The research that has produced this book lends support to the public health side of this debate, but with an important qualification.

The important thing in public health is not the technical knowledge and skill of the experts who give advice about disease prevention. It is instead the participation of ordinary people in the effort.

The third element in the plan for development is thus for people to discover that they can be engaged in controlling health risks. This is the essential point: people can be counted on to become allies and participants in social growth and improving health.

Chronology of Health Transitions and Gross Domestic Product per Capita (GDPpc) in 167 Countries

Period[1]	Country	Life Expectancy at Initiation of Health Transition[2]	Life Expectancy in 2000	GDPpc at Initiation of Health Transition (1990 international dollars)	GDPpc in 2000 (1990 international dollars)
1770s (1775)	Denmark	c. 33	76.4	1,186[3]	23,010
1790s (1795)	France	28.1	78.6	1,088[3]	20,808
	Sweden	35.3 (1781–90)	79.7	1,152[3]	20,321
1800s (1805)	England	36.3 (1796–1805)	77.7 (1998–2000, England and Wales)	2,006 (England, Wales, and Scotland)	19,817 (UK)
1810s (1815)	Norway	38.3 (1801–15)	78.6	1,104	24,364
1820s or 1830s (1830)	Canada	39.0	78.9	904	22,198
1840s (1845)	Belgium	38.3 (1843–50)	78.4	1,694	20,742
1820s to 1890s (1860)	Ireland	38.3 (1821–41)	76.3	1,775	22,015

1860s or 1870s (1870)	Australia[4]	48.0	78.9	3,273	21,540
	Netherlands	37.3 (1850–59)	77.9	2,757	21,591
	New Zealand[4]	51.8–53.1 (1870s)	78.2	3,100	16,010
1860s to 1900s (1890)	Mexico	24–29	73.0	1,189	7,218
1870s (1875)	Finland	32.1	77.5	1,211	20,235
	Germany	36.7–38.4	77.4	2,112	18,596
	Iceland	32.3	79.5	n.a.	n.a.
	Switzerland	40.3–40.7 (1876–78)	80.3	2,645	22,025
	UK: Scotland	42.1 (1860s)	75.4	2,006 (England, Wales, and Scotland	19,817 (UK)
1870s or 1880s (1880)	Italy	35.4 (1881–82)	78.7	1,581	18,740
	Luxembourg	n.a.	77.0	n.a.	n.a.
1870s to 1890s (1890)	Japan	36.6 (1870)	80.7	1,012	21,069
1880s (1885)	Poland	n.a.	73.3	1,284 (1890)	7,215
	United States	39.4 (1880; 40.5, whites only)	77.1	3,106	28,129
1880s or 1890s (1890)	Austria	31.7 (1865–75)	78.2	2,443	20,097
	Hungary	n.a.	71.3	1,473	7,138
1890s (1895)	Czech Republic	35	74.8	1,617	9,047
	Slovak Republic	n.a.	73.1	1,617	7,837
	Spain	29.5 (1878–87)	78.2	1,689	15,269
1890s or 1900s (1900)	Argentina	33.3	73.9	2,756	8,544
	Cyprus	38.5 (1890s)	77.9	n.a.	n.a.

	Russia	31 (1897)	65.3	1,237	5,157
1890s to 1920s (1890)	Costa Rica	30.5 (1890s) 33.3–34.1 (1920s)	77.5	1,624 (1920)	6,174
(1920)	Estonia	43.1 (c. 1900)	70.6	n.a.	n.a.
(1920)	Latvia	45 (1896–97)	70.4	n.a.	n.a.
(1920)	Lithuania	41.7 (c. 1900)	72.6	n.a.	n.a.
(1920)	Ukraine	36.6 (c. 1900)	68.3	n.a.	2,736
1900s (1905)	Cuba	33.1–38.4	76.5	n.a.	2,414
	Puerto Rico	30.4–32.1 (1894)	76.1	n.a.	14,106
1900s or 1910s (1910)	Greece	38–40	77.9	1,592 (1913)	12,044
1900s to 1920s (1920)	Singapore	n.a.	77.7	1,279 (1913)	22,207
	Yugoslavia	n.a.	72.5	1,031	4,258
1910s (1915)	Korea	23.5	73.2 (South) 60.7 (North)	966	14,343 (South)
	Panama	n.a.	74.6	n.a.	5,782
1910s or 1920s (1920)	Romania	n.a.	69.9	1,258 (1926)	3,002
1910s to 1930s (1930)	Malaysia	n.a.	72.5	1,636	7,872
	Philippines	25.6–37.5 (1918)	69.3	1,476	2,385
1920s (1925)	Bangladesh	24.9 (1921–31)	61.2	n.a.	873
	Bulgaria	44.6	71.6	922	5,365
	Chile	31.6	75.7	2,876	9,841
	China	24.2–35	70.3	562 (1929)	3,425
	Fiji	n.a.	69.2	n.a.	n.a.
	Ghana	28	56.9	n.a.	1,280
	Guyana	31.1 (1911)	62.9	n.a.	n.a.
	India	24.9	62.8	698	1,910

	Indonesia	30	66.0	1,010	3,203
	Jamaica	37.0	75.3	789[3]	3,548
	Mauritius	31.2	71.7	n.a.	n.a.
	Pakistan	20.1 (1921)	63.0	n.a.	1,920
	Portugal	n.a.	75.7	n.a.	14,022
	Sri Lanka	29.9 (1911)	73.1	1,187	3,645
	Suriname	n.a.	70.2	n.a.	n.a.
	Taiwan	30.8 (1911–20)	76.4	1,099	16,642
	Trinidad and Tobago	39.4	72.6	n.a.	13,598
	Tunisia	28.8	72.1	n.a.	4,538
	Uruguay	50.0	74.4	3,188	7,859
1920s or 1930s (1930)	Albania	less than 38.3	74.0	n.a.	2,807
	Brazil	32.0	68.1	1,048	5,556
	Paraguay	26.1 (1899)	70.4	1,894 (1939)	3,014
	South Africa	n.a.	47.8	n.a.	4,139
	Turkey	n.a.	69.7	n.a.	6,597
	Venezuela	32.2 (1926)	73.4	3,444	8,415
	Vietnam	22.5	69.1	n.a.	n.a.
1930s (1935)	Algeria	31.2	71.0	n.a.	2,792
	Colombia	32–40	71.6	1,677	5,096
	Egypt	31–32	67.5	n.a.	2,920
	Guatemala	25.8	65.2	1,712	3,396
	Jordan	n.a.	71.5	n.a.	4,055
	Kenya	23.9	47	n.a.	1,020
	Syria	n.a.	69.7	n.a.	7,481
	Uganda	23.9	42.1	n.a.	788
1930s or 1940s (1940)	Bolivia	25.5 (1900)	62.6	1,690 (1945)	2,575
	Congo Democratic Republic	n.a.	45.8	570 (1950)	218
	Dominican Republic	29.9	67.3	n.a.	3,663
	Ecuador	n.a.	69.6	1,356	3,101
	El Salvador	28.7	70.2	1,111	2,716
	Honduras	33.9 (1930)	66.0	1,160	1,957

	Iran	25 (1926)	69.1	1,720 (1950)	4,911
	Iraq	n.a.	61.1	1,364 (1950)	1,294
	Kuwait	26	76.6	28,878 (1950)	10,115
	Laos	n.a.	53.7	n.a.	n.a.
	Lebanon	n.a.	70.4	2,429 (1950)	3,430
	Libya	42.9 (1950)	71.0	857 (1950)	2,322
	Morocco	n.a.	67.5	1,455 (1950)	2,658
	Namibia	31.3–38.7 (1950)	47.2	2,160 (1950)	3,795
	Nicaragua	24.4 (1921)	68.9	1,372	1,558
	Peru	36.4 (1940)	69.3	1,823	3,686
	Qatar	n.a.	74.8	30,387 (1950)	8,268
	Senegal	23.9–36.4	52.3	1,259 (1950)	1,433
	Sudan	n.a.	56.2	821 (1950)	991
	Thailand	38.3–40.3	68.8	826 (1938)	6,336
	United Arab Emirates	n.a.	75.3	15,798 (1950)	16,560
	Zimbabwe	26.4 (mid-1930s)	39.9	701 (1950)	1,280
1930s to 1950s (1950)	Burundi	c. 31	42.0	360	575
	Cape Verde	n.a.	68.8	450	1,777
	Myanmar	30.8 (1926)	56.1	396	1,353
	Rwanda	33.5 (1950) and 39 (1970)	39.9	547	830
1940s (1945)	Bahrain	n.a.	73.1	2,104 (1950)	5,065
	Lesotho	35.9 (1950)	44.0	355 (1950)	1,645
	Papua New Guinea	31.5 (1946)	58.6	n.a.	n.a.

	Sierra Leone	24.5 (1931)	39.2	656 (1950)	379
	Solomon Islands	44.0 (1950–55)	68.6	n.a.	n.a.
1940s or 1950s (1950)	Afghanistan	30.2	43.0	n.a.	n.a.
	Angola	27.0	46.6	1,052	789
	Benin	c. 31	53.0	1,084	1,323
	Botswana	c. 33	39.0	349	4,348
	Burkina Faso	c. 31	44.2	474	853
	Cambodia	35 or less	53.8	n.a.	n.a.
	Cameroon	28.8 (1931); 33.5 (1950)	50.1	671	1,115
	Central African Rep.	c. 33	43.5	772	647
	Chad	c. 30	48.5	476	424
	Comoros	n.a.	60.7	560	581
	Congo Republic	c. 32	51.3	1,289	2,214
	Cote d'Ivoire	c. 32	45.8	1,041	1,326
	Djibouti	c. 33	45.8	1,500	1,103
	Equatorial Guinea	c. 34	49.1	540	7,956
	Eritrea	n.a.	51.0	390	624
	Ethiopia	c. 30	42.3	390	624
	Gabon	c. 31	52.7	3,108	3,887
	Gambia	30–33.5	53.3	607	895
	Guinea	c. 31	46.3	303	572
	Guinea Bissau	c. 28	44.9	289	681
	Haiti	n.a.	53.2	n.a.	810
	Liberia	34.5 (1950)	47.2	1,055	847
	Madagascar	33.5 (1950)	54.7	951	706
	Malawi	33.5 (1950)	38.8	324	679
	Mali	33.5 (1950)	42.3	457	842
	Mauritania	33.5 (1950)	51.7	464	1,017
	Mongolia	42.2–45 (1950–55)	67.0	n.a.	n.a.
	Nepal	33.1 (1950)	58.9	496	999

	Niger	33.5 (1950)	45.7	813	503
	Nigeria	20–32 (1931)	46.8	753	1,156
	Saudi Arabia	30–34.5	72.5	2,231	8,002
	Somalia	33–33.5 (1950)	48.1	1,057	863
	Swaziland	33.4 (1950)	45.6	721	2,606
	Tanzania	34.2 (1950)	44.4	424	524
	Togo	31.3 (1950)	49.3	574	575
	Yemen	34.7 (1950)	56.5	911	2,588
	Zambia	36 (1950)	38.0	661	666
1940s to 1970s (1965)	Mozambique	32–33.5 (1950)	42.4	1,364	1,432
	Oman	40.3 (1960)	73.6	1,053	6,926

SOURCES: Angus Maddison, *The World Economy: Historical Statistics* (Paris: Development Center of the Organization for Economic Cooperation and Development, 2003); James C. Riley, "The Timing and Pace of Health Transitions around the World," *Population and Development Review* 31 (2005): 758–62.

1. Dates in parentheses in the first column indicate the year used for interpolating between Maddison's GDPpc estimates to arrive at a figure at the initiation of a country's health transition.

2. A range of figures for life expectancy estimates signals that information has been taken from two or more sources that provide different figures.

3. By straight line interpolation.

4. Sustained gains date from the periods indicated, but in both cases most of the in-migrating population came from areas where mortality had begun to decline before migration to the South Pacific began. Thus Australia and New Zealand are not strictly similar to most cases listed here.

Notes

Preface and Acknowledgments

1. United Nations Development Programme, *Human Development Report 2004* (New York: Oxford University Press, 2004), p. 139, for 2002.

Introduction

1. P. G. K. Panikar, "Fall in Mortality Rates in Kerala: An Explanatory Hypothesis," *Economic and Political Weekly* 10 (1975): 1811–18; Panikar, "Resources Not the Constraint on Health Improvement: A Case Study of Kerala," *Economic and Political Weekly* 14 (1979): 1803–9; and John Ratcliffe, "Social Justice and the Demographic Transition: Lessons from India's Kerala State," *International Journal of Health Services* 8 (1978): 123–44.

2. John C. Caldwell, "Routes to Low Mortality in Poor Countries," *Population and Development Review* 12 (1986): 171–220. This remains one of the most widely cited articles in the field of demography. See the Web of Knowledge's cited reference search at www.isiwebofknowledge.com.

3. Scott B. Halstead, Julia A. Walsh, and Kenneth S. Warren, eds., *Good Health at Low Cost* (New York: Rockefeller Foundation, 1985). See also Godfrey Gunatilleke, ed., *Intersectoral Linkages and Health Development: Case Studies in India (Kerala State), Jamaica, Norway, Sri Lanka, and Thailand* (Geneva: World Health Organization, 1984), which concentrates on the disease clusters typical at different levels of development and recommends "the active involvement of the health sector in social development planning" (p. 48) and the development of "health consciousness" (p. 49) in the population, among other ideas.

4. Dharam Ghai, ed., *Social Development and Public Policy: A Study of Some Successful Experiences* (Houndmills, Hampshire, U.K.: Macmillan, 2000), quotes from pp. ix–x. For Ghai's summary of common findings, see pp. 1–45.

5. Santosh Mehrotra, "Integrating Economic and Social Policy: Good Practices from High-Achieving Countries," Innocenti Working Paper No. 80, 2000; and Santosh Mehrotra and Richard Jolly, eds., *Development with a Human Face: Experiences in Social Achievement and Economic Growth* (Oxford: Clarendon Press, 1997). The quote comes from Mehrotra, "Social Development in High-Achieving Countries: Common Elements and Diversities," in *Development with a Human Face*, p. 32. See also Amartya Sen, *Development as Freedom* (New York: Knopf, 1999), pp. 46–49.

6. James C. Riley, "Estimates of Regional and Global Life Expectancy, 1800–2000," *Population and Development Review* 31 (2005): 537–43; and Riley, "The Timing and Pace of Health Transitions around the World," *Population and Development Review* 31 (2005): 741–64. See also the list of works consulted for these studies in James C. Riley, "Bibliography of Works Providing Estimates of Life Expectancy at Birth and of the Beginning Period of Health Transitions in Countries with a Population in 2000 of at least 400,000" at www.lifetable.de/Riley Bib.htm, with comments on sources preferred for certain estimates.

7. Thomas McKeown, *The Modern Rise of Population* (London: Edward Arnold, 1976). McKeown also related his findings to some other countries in Thomas McKeown, R. G. Brown, and R. G. Record, "An Interpretation of the Modern Rise of Population in Europe," *Population Studies* 26 (1972): 345–82.

8. Peter H. Lindert, *Growing Public: Social Spending and Economic Growth since the Eighteenth Century,* 2 vols. (Cambridge: Cambridge University Press, 2004), 1: 171–90; and Lindert, "The Rise of Social Spending, 1880–1930," *Explorations in Economic History* 31 (1994): 1–37.

9. Arthur Livingstone, *Social Policy in Developing Countries* (London: Routledge and K. Paul, 1969), quote from p. 8.

10. See James C. Riley, *Rising Life Expectancy: A Global History* (Cambridge: Cambridge University Press, 2001), chapters 2, 3, and 7 for a more detailed treatment about how public health, medicine, and education have influenced health.

11. Majid Ezzati et al., "Estimates of Global and Regional Potential Health Gains from Reducing Multiple Major Risk Factors," *The Lancet* 362 (July 26, 2003): 271–80.

12. Sweden is an exception. There infant mortality declined across the nineteenth century.

13. E.g., the United States, on which see David Cutler and Grant Miller, "The Role of Public Health Improvements in Health Advances: The Twentieth-Century United States," *Demography* 42 (2005): 1–22.

14. For a recent literature review and introduction to the standard of living debate, see Jane Humphries, "Standard of Living, Quality of Life," in *A Companion to Nineteenth-Century Britain,* ed. Chris Williams (Malden, MA: Blackwell, 2004), pp. 287–304. And for a new interpretation of the health problems created by economic growth, see Simon Szreter, *Health and Wealth: Studies in History and Policy* (Rochester: University of Rochester Press, 2005), pp. 416–47.

15. Philip D. Curtin, *Death by Migration: Europe's Encounter with the Tropical World in the Nineteenth Century* (Cambridge: Cambridge University Press, 1989), p. 160; and Curtin, *Disease and Empire: The Health of European Troops in the Conquest of Africa* (Cambridge: Cambridge University Press, 1998), p. 229.

16. Because the information used to gauge income distribution has been collected in different ways in different countries, it is sometimes difficult to make valid comparisons across time in the same country and always difficult to make such comparisons across countries. In general, recent estimates, those dealing with the period since the 1950s, are likelier to allow comparisons that are sufficiently accurate.

17. C. Morrison, "Historical Perspectives on Income Distribution: The Case of Europe," in *Handbook of Income Distribution,* ed. Anthony B. Atkinson and François Bourguignon (Amsterdam: Elsevier, 2000), pp. 225–28; and Johan Söderberg, "Wage Differentials in Sweden, 1725–1950," in *Income Distribution in Historical Perspective,* ed. Y. S. Brenner, Hartmut Kaelble, and Mark Thomas (Cambridge: Cambridge University Press, 1991), pp. 76–95.

18. For the case that uneven income distribution impedes survival, see Nancy E. Adler et al., eds., *Socioeconomic Status and Health in Industrial Nations: Social, Psychological, and Biological Pathways,* vol. 896 of *Annals of the New York Academy of Sciences* (New York: New York Academy of Science, 1999); James A. Auerbach and Barbara Kivinae Krimgold, eds., *Income, Socioeconomic Status, and Health: Exploring the Relationships* (Washington: National Policy Association and Academy for Health Services Research and Health Policy, 2001); and Richard Wilkinson, *Unhealthy Societies: The Afflictions of Inequality* (London: Routledge, 1996), pp. 34–36. (See chapter 3 for discussion of Wilkinson's treatment of Japan.) However, John Lynch et al., "Is Income Inequality a Determinant of Population Health? Part 1. A Systematic Review," *Milbank Quarterly* 82 (2004): 5–99, review evidence from a large number of studies and find little support for this idea. So, too, Jason Beckfield, "Does Income Inequality Harm Health? New Cross-National Evidence," *Journal of Health and Social Behavior* 45 (2004): 231–48.

19. Gretchen A. Condran and Samuel H. Preston, "Child Mortality Differences, Personal Health Practices, and Medical Technology: The United States, 1900–1930," in *Health and Social Change in International Perspective,* ed. Lincoln Chen, Arthur Kleinman, and Norma C. Ware (Boston: Department of Population and International Health, Harvard School of Public Health, 1993), pp. 171–224; and Samuel H. Preston and Michael R. Haines, *Fatal Years: Child Mortality in Late Nineteenth-Century America* (Princeton: Princeton University Press, 1991), esp. pp. 171, 175.

1. Life Expectancy and Income among the First Countries to Begin Health Transitions

1. James C. Riley, "Estimates of Regional and Global Life Expectancy, 1800–2000," *Population and Development Review* 31 (2005): 537–43; and Riley, "The Timing and Pace of Health Transitions around the World," *Population and Development Review* 31 (2005): 741–64.

2. These estimates exclude the European populations of Australia and New Zealand, most of which migrated from countries where health transitions had already begun.

3. This value is unweighted by population.

4. Gy. Acsádi and J. Nemeskéri, *History of Human Life Span and Mortality,* trans. K. Balás (Budapest: Akadémiai Kiadó, 1970).

5. Interestingly, French life expectancy in parts of the eighteenth century was as low as that in Neolithic populations in North Africa. See ibid., pp. 160, 205, 266–67, and 282–83; and Yves Blayo, "La mortalité en France de 1740 à 1829," *Population,* Special Number 30 (1975): 123–42.

6. There are exceptions, with varying lengths. In the British West Indies survival in the African-background population rose from the end of slavery in the 1830s until at least the 1860s but that increase did not persist. Campbell reports a long period of rising life expectancy in the Qing imperial lineage from the mid-seventeenth to the late nineteenth century, which was then interrupted. Hayami finds persistent decline in crude death rates in his study of towns in Japan from the 1670s to the 1860s. See G. W. Roberts, "A Life Table for a West Indian Slave Population," *Population Studies* 5 (1951–52): 238–43; James C. Riley, *Poverty and Life Expectancy: The Jamaica Paradox* (Cambridge: Cambridge University Press, 2005), pp. 23–25; Cameron Campbell, "Mortality Change and the Epidemiological Transition in Beijing, 1644–1990," in *Asian Population History,* ed. Ts'ui-jung Liu et al. (Oxford: Oxford University Press, 2001), pp. 221–47; and Akira Hayami, *The Historical Demography of Pre-Modern Japan* (Tokyo: University of Tokyo Press, 2001), pp. 88–89.

7. Gustav Sundbärg, *Bevölkerungsstatistik Schwedens 1750–1900* (Stockholm: Statistiska Centralbyrån, 1970), p. 158.

8. Peter Sköld, *The Two Faces of Smallpox: A Disease and Its Prevention in Eighteenth- and Nineteenth-Century Sweden* (Umeå: Demographic Data Base, Umeå University, 1996), pp. 52, 388–422, and 449, quote from 443.

9. Phyllis Deane, *Colonial Social Accounting* (Cambridge: Cambridge University Press, 1953), pp. 22–25 and 115–30, quotes from p. xiv.

10. Claremont P. Kirton, "Informal Economic Activities in Selected Caribbean Countries," unpublished paper, March 1991; and Michael Witter and Claremont Kirton, "The Informal Economy in Jamaica: Some Empirical Exercises," ISER Working Paper No. 36, 1990.

11. Janet MacGaffey et al., *The Real Economy of Zaire: The Contribution of Smuggling and Other Unofficial Activities to National Wealth* (Philadelphia: University of Pennsylvania Press, 1991), p. 11.

12. Edward Smithies, *The Black Economy in England since 1914* (Dublin: Gill and Macmillan, 1984), esp. pp. 3–4, 129–31.

13. Angus Maddison, *The World Economy: Historical Statistics* (Paris: Development Center of the Organization for Economic Cooperation and Development, 2003), pp. 87 and 218–23.

14. Calculated from information obtained at the Bureau of Labor website, www.bls.gov/cpi/home.htm, accessed July 10, 2005.

15. Maddison's estimates are contentious, no less for 1820 than for other periods. Some historians believe China was much richer, in comparison to Europe; others suggest that the United States may have been the richest land in the world around 1790. But the disparities that Maddison estimates across countries seem roughly appropriate. So, too, does the European hierarchy, keeping in mind that England is embedded within Great Britain.

16. The group of fourteen cases includes two (England and northern Italy) for which life expectancy estimates are for smaller regions than are the GDPpc estimates. Dropping these two cases produces an adjusted R-square of 0.048 and a significance level of 0.241.

17. The seven early-transition countries not included in table 2 are Iceland, Scotland, and Cyprus (no GDPpc); Poland, Hungary, and the Slovak Republic (no life expectancy figure); and Luxembourg (neither data point available).

18. Indeed the United States and the Netherlands may have done so. For both, urbanization and high levels of mortality in cities may mask earlier beginning periods.

19. Including other countries for 1870 or 1913 would presumably elevate the adjusted R-square value since most of those countries could have been low-income and low life expectancy cases.

20. With fewer data pairs, Samuel H. Preston, "The Changing Relation between Mortality and Level of Economic Development," *Population Studies* 29 (1975): 231–48, found an almost equally strong correlation in the 1930s and the 1960s but a changing ratio of income and life expectancy, and suggested that the relationship was shifting by the early 1900s. Specifically, he found that the income level necessary to allow a life expectancy between 40 and 60 years dropped between the 1900s and the 1930, and again between the 1930s and the 1960s. See also United Nations, *Levels and Trends of Mortality since 1950* (New York: United Nations, Department of International Economic and Social Affairs, 1982), pp. 38–42.

Among studies whose authors are impressed by the association in the late twentieth century, see Griffith Feeney and Andrew Mason, "Population in East Asia," in *Population Change and Economic Development in East Asia: Challenges Met, Opportunities Seized,* ed. Andrew Mason (Stanford, CA: Stanford University Press, 2001), pp. 61–95; and Lant Pritchett and Lawrence H. Summers, "Wealthier Is Healthier," *Journal of Human Resources* 31 (1996): 841–68.

21. For explorations of this idea see Suchit Arora, "Health, Human Productivity, and Long-Term Economic Growth," *Journal of Economic History* 61 (2001): 699–749; and Robert Barro, "Determinants of Economic Growth: A Cross-Country Empirical Study," National Bureau of Economic Research Working Paper 5698, 1997.

22. The adjusted R- square equals 0.296 and is statistically significant at the 0.01 level. Current levels of life expectancy and health spending are of course functions of historical processes.

23. Alan Macfarlane, *The Savage Wars of Peace: England, Japan and the Malthusian Trap* (Oxford: Blackwell, 1997).

2. Which Countries Should Be Studied?

1. Jia Wang et al., *Measuring Country Performance on Health: Selected Indicators for 115 Countries* (Washington: World Bank, 1999), identify underachieving and overachieving countries in the period 1960–90, but they avoid asking why particular countries occupied the positions they observe.

2. The sources for this database are listed at James C. Riley, "Bibliography of

Works Providing Estimates of Life Expectancy at Birth and of the Beginning Period of Health Transitions in Countries with a Population in 2000 of at least 400,000" at www.lifetable.de/RileyBib.htm, with comments on sources preferred for certain estimates. See also Riley, "Estimates of Regional and Global Life Expectancy, 1800–2000," *Population and Development Review* 31 (2005): 537–43; and "The Timing and Pace of Health Transitions around the World," *Population and Development Review* 31 (2005): 741–64.

3. José Miguel Avilán Rovira, "Situación de salud en Venezuela según las estadísticas de mortalidad 1940–1995," *Gaceta médica de Caracas* 106 (1998): 169–96; see p. 185.

4. Ann Jannetta, "Public Health and the Diffusion of Vaccination in Japan," unpublished paper, International Union for the Scientific Study of Population, 1996.

5. Charles W. LeBaron and David W. Taylor, "Typhoid Fever," in *The Cambridge World History of Human Disease,* ed. Kenneth F. Kiple (Cambridge: Cambridge University Press, 1993), pp. 1071–77, quote from p. 1074. The protection was also not permanent. For details and more recent refinements, see Myron M. Levine, "Typhoid Fever Vaccines," in *Vaccines,* ed. Stanley A. Plotkin and Walter A. Orenstein, 4th ed. (Philadelphia: W. B. Saunders, 2004), pp. 1057–93.

6. James C. Riley, *Poverty and Life Expectancy: The Jamaica Paradox* (Cambridge: Cambridge University Press, 2005), p. 113.

7. On the timing of new vaccines, see especially the articles in Stanley A. Plotkin and Edward A. Mortimer, Jr., eds., *Vaccines,* 2nd ed. (Philadelphia: W. B. Saunders, 1994).

3. A Colonizer and the Country Colonized

1. Estimates of GDPpc and life expectancy refer to all of the Korean peninsula until about 1950, and from the mid 1950s to South Korea (Republic of Korea).

2. Regarding Japan, Haruo Mizushima, "Reformation of Early Life Tables for Japan," *Minzoku Eisei* 28 (1962): 64–74, and Chotaro Takahashi, Ryotaro Iochi, and Koichi Emi, *Dynamic Changes of Income and Its Distribution in Japan* (Tokyo: Kinokuniya Bookstore Co., 1959), report an increase in life expectancy and a decrease in infant mortality in the period 1870–1913. Others suggest instead that infant mortality did not decrease until the 1920s, when it fell sharply. See Osamu Saito, *Infant Mortality in Pre-Transition Japan: Levels and Trends* (Tokyo: Institute of Economic Research, Hitotsubashi University, 1993); Saito, "Infant Mortality in Pre-Transition Japan: Levels and Trends," in *Infant and Child Mortality in the Past,* eds. Alain Bideau, Bertrand Desjardins, and Héctor Pérez Brignoli (Oxford: Oxford University Press, 1997), pp. 135–53; and Masato Takase, "Vital Rates and Population Statistics of Japan, 1890–1920," *Jinkogaku kenkyu* 14 (1991): 21–34 (in Japanese; Hiromi Yampol translated this material for me.)

See also Akíra Hayami, *The Historical Demography of Pre-Modern Japan* (Tokyo: University of Tokyo Press, 2001); Ann Bowman Jannetta and Samuel H. Preston, "Two Centuries of Mortality Change in Central Japan: The Evidence from a Tem-ple Death Register," *Population Studies* 45 (1991): 417–36; and S. Ryan Johansson and Carl Mosk, "Exposure, Resistance and Life Expectancy: Disease and Death during the Economic Development of Japan, 1900–1960," *Population Studies* 41 (1987): 207–35.

3. Machiko Yanagishita and Jack M. Guralnik, "Changing Mortality Patterns That Led Life Expectancy in Japan to Surpass Sweden's: 1971–1982," *Demography* 25 (1988): 611–24.

4. Susan B. Hanley, "Fertility, Mortality, and Life Expectancy in Pre-Modern Japan," *Population Studies* 28 (1974): 127–42; Hanley, "A High Standard of Living in Nineteenth-Century Japan: Fact or Fantasy?" *Journal of Economic History* 43 (1983): 183–92; Hanley, "Urban Sanitation in Preindustrial Japan," *Journal of Interdisciplinary History* 18 (1987): 1–26; and Alan Macfarlane, *The Savage Wars of Peace: England, Japan and the Malthusian Trap* (Oxford: Blackwell, 1997). Estimates for the influenza epidemic of 1918–19 are unavailable.

5. Toshiyuki Mizoguchi and Noriyuki Takayama, *Equity and Poverty under Rapid Economic Growth: The Japanese Experience* (Tokyo: Kinokuniya Co., 1984), pp. 215–16, quote from p. 216.

6. Naoko T. Miyaji and Margaret Lock, "Monitoring Motherhood: Sociocultural and Historical Aspects of Maternal and Child Health in Japan," *Daedalus* 123 (1994): 87–112; Yonezo Nakagawa, "Adoption of Western Medicine in Japan," *Clio Medica* 21 (1987–88): 113–18; and F. Ohtani, ed., *One Hundred Years of Health Progress in Japan* (Tokyo: International Medical Foundation of Japan, 1971).

7. Japan, Ministry of Health and Welfare, *A Brief Report on Public Health Administration in Japan* (Tokyo: n.p., 1970); and Irene B. Taeuber, *The Population of Japan* (Princeton: Princeton University Press, 1958), p. 286.

8. Samuel H. Preston, Nathan Keyfitz, and Robert Schoen, *Causes of Death: Life Tables for National Populations* (New York: Seminar Press, 1972), pp. 420–23; and Taeuber, *Population of Japan,* p. 290.

9. Taeuber, *Population of Japan,* p. 284 nn. 1, 2.

10. Japan also set a strict standard of sanitation and hygiene for its troops in the Russo-Japanese War of 1904–5 and reduced the ratio of deaths from disease to battle deaths. See Louis Livingston Seaman, *The Real Triumph of Japan: The Conquest of the Silent Foe* (New York: Appleton, 1908).

11. Michael D. Stephens, *Japan and Education* (London: St. Martin's Press, 1991), pp. 34–35.

12. Mikiso Hane, *Peasants, Rebels, and Outcastes: The Underside of Modern Japan* (New York: Pantheon, 1982), p. 51.

13. Miyaji and Lock, "Monitoring Motherhood." The 1872 Regulations for Primary Schools called for two hours instruction weekly in hygiene in each of the third, fourth, and fifth years of primary school, which the 1881 regulations replaced with physiology at a higher level. Japan, Ministry of Education, *The Role of Education in the Social and Economic Development of Japan* (Tokyo: Institute for Democratic Education, 1966), pp. 53 and 57.

14. Koji Taira, "Education and Literacy in Meiji Japan: An Interpretation," *Explorations in Economic History* 8 (1971): 371–94.

15. G. Balatchandirane, "Role of Education in Japan's Modernisation: A Reassessment," *China Report* 31 (1995): 219–33.

16. Kumiko Fujimura-Fanselow, "The Japanese Ideology of 'Good Wives and Wise Mothers': Trends in Contemporary Research," *Gender and History* 3 (1991): 345–49.

17. David R. Ambaras, "Social Knowledge, Cultural Capital, and the New Middle Class in Japan, 1895–1912," *Journal of Japanese Studies* 24 (1998): 1–33.

18. Angus Maddison, *The World Economy: Historical Statistics* (Paris: Development Center of the Organization for Economic Cooperation and Development, 2003), pp. 60–61 and 180.

19. A. Radha Krishnan and Malcolm Tull, "Resource Use and Environmental Management in Japan, 1890–1990," *Australian Economic History Review* 34 (1994): 3–23.

20. United Nations Development Programme, World Income Inequality Database, available at www.wider.unu.edu/wiid/wwwwiid.htm, citing Toshiyuki Mizoguchi, "Economic Development Policy and Income Distribution: The Experience in East and Southeast Asia," *The Developing Economies* 23 (1985): 307–24.

21. On the prewar period see also K. Aoki, "The Changing Health Spectrum in Japan: Facts and Implications," in *New Developments in the Analysis of Mortality and Causes of Death,* ed. Harald Hansluwka et al. (Bangkok: Faculty of Public Health, Institute for Population and Social Research, Mahidol University, 1986), pp. 409–36; and Ohtani, ed., *One Hundred Years of Health Progress.*

22. On the postwar period, in addition to sources cited below, see Itsuzo Shigematsu and Masaki Nagai, "Factors Associated with the Decline of Mortality in Japan," in *Mortality in South and East Asia: A Review of Changing Trends and Patterns, 1950–1975* (Manila: World Health Organization, 1982); and Takao Shigematsu, *Factors Contributing to the Improvement and Predominance of the Longevity of the Japanese Population* (Tokyo: Nihon University, Population Research Institute, 1994).

23. Aoki, "Changing Health Spectrum in Japan," pp. 409–36; and Yoshiyuki Ohno, "Health Development in Japan: Determinants, Implications and Perspectives," *World Health Statistics Quarterly* 38 (1985): 176–92. On links between survival gains in the 1950s and 1960s and later gains, see K. Yoshinaga and H. Une, "Contributions of Mortality Changes by Age Group and Selected Causes of Death to the Increase in Japanese Life Expectancy at Birth from 1950 to 2000," *European Journal of Epidemiology* 20 (2005): 49–57.

24. Shinsuke Morio and Shigesato Takahashi, "Socio-economic Correlates of Mortality in Japan," in *Socio-Economic Correlates of Mortality in Japan and ASEAN,* ed. Shui Meng Ng (Singapore: Institute of Southeast Asian Studies, 1986), pp. 18–61, report that differing ratios of population covered by the water supply system continued to show a statistical association with high infant mortality as late as 1980.

25. Eikichi Matsuyama, *Saving the Children: How Japan Keeps Down Its Infant Mortality Rate* (Tokyo: Japanese Organization for International Cooperation in Family Planning, 1986).

26. T. Shigematsu, *Factors Contributing to . . . Longevity*.

27. Maddison, *World Economy*, pp. 63, 65, and 184.

28. The proportion of the population living in cities jumped from 28 percent in 1945 to 63 percent in 1960. Toshio Kuroda et al., *Urbanization and Development in Japan* (Tokyo: Asian Population and Development Association, 1986), p. 26.

29. UNDP, World Income Inequality Database, citing Toshiyuki Mizoguchi and Noriyuki Takayama, *Equity and Poverty under Rapid Economic Growth: The Japanese Experience* (Tokyo: Kinokuniya Co., 1984). Chiaki Moriguchi and Emmanuel Saez, "The Evolution of Income Concentration in Japan, 1885–2002: Evidence from Income Tax Statistics," unpublished paper, version dated August 14, 2004, report that the concentration of income toward the top of the distribution dropped during and after World War II and then remained relatively stable from 1951 to 2002.

30. Assessments may consider income or net income after taxation and transfers from such sources as pensions. States with low Gini coefficients usually achieve that position by using taxation and government spending to equalize the distribution of income or consumption.

31. Anthony B. Atkinson, Lee Rainwater, and Timothy M. Smeeding, *Income Distribution in OECD Countries: Evidence from the Luxembourg Income Study* (Paris: Organization for Economic Cooperation and Development, 1995), p. 46.

32. G. B. Rodgers, "Income and Inequality as Determinants of Mortality: An International Cross-Section Analysis," *Population Studies* 33 (1979): 343–51, quote from p. 350.

33. Richard Wilkinson, *Unhealthy Societies: The Afflictions of Inequality* (London: Routledge, 1996), quotes from p. 7. The argument is developed further in Michael Marmot and Richard G. Wilkinson, eds., *Social Determinants of Health* (Oxford: Oxford University Press, 1999); and many essays pertinent to this argument are collected in Ichiro Kawachi, Bruce P. Kennedy, and Richard G. Wilkinson, eds., *The Society and Population Health Reader*, vol. 1 (New York: New Press, 1999; additional volumes planned). See note 18 to the introduction for sources critiquing this interpretation.

34. Wilkinson, *Unhealthy Societies*, pp. 130–34. See also M. G. Marmot and George Davey Smith, "Why Are the Japanese Living Longer?" *British Journal of Medicine* 299 (1989): 1547–51.

35. Wilkinson, *Unhealthy Societies*, p. 130.

36. See the comparative data available in the UNDP World Income Inequality Database, accessed December 23, 2004.

37. Yunshik Chang, "Population in Early Modernization: Korea" (PhD diss., Princeton University, 1967), pp. 201–10 and 263ff; Doo-Sub Kim and Cheong-Seok Kim, eds., *The Population of Korea* (Daejeon: Korean National Statistical Office, 2004), pp. 93–94; Tai-Hun Kim, *Mortality Transition in Korea 1960–1980* (Seoul: Population and Development Studies Center, Seoul National University, 1990), p. 146; Tai-Hwan Kwon, *Demography of Korea: Population Change and Its Components, 1925–66* (Seoul: Seoul National University Press, 1977); Tai-Hwan Kwon, *The Trends and Patterns of Mortality and Health in the Republic of Korea* (Bangkok: Economic

and Social Commission for Asia and the Pacific, 1986); Eun-Sul Lee, "Epidemiologic Transition in Korea: A New Perspective in Population and Development Studies," *Bulletin of the Population and Development Studies Center* 14 (1985): 1–14; and Hae-Young Lee, "Demographic Transition in Korea," *Bulletin of the Population and Development Studies Center* 8 and 9 (1980): 5–17. Death registration improved during the colonial period, 1910–45, but remained incomplete into the 1960s. Thus scholars debate the survival level in each period, especially during the 1950s.

38. Chang, *Population in Early Modernization,* pp. 282–90; T.-H. Kwon, *Demography of Korea,* pp. 53–55. Also Yoshikuni Ishi, *Kankoku no jinko zoka no bunseki* [An analysis of population growth in Korea] (Tokyo: Keiso Shobo, 1972), who dates mortality decline from the mid-1930s. (Hiromi Yampol translated Ishi's book for me.) On causes of death see E-Hyock Kwon and Tae-Ryong Kim, "The Population of Korea," *Journal of Population Studies* 7 (1968): 157–59.

39. Sherwood Hall, *With Stethoscope in Asia: Korea* (McLean, VA: MCL Associates, 1978), pp. 148–50, 388, and 436; quote from p. 367.

40. Mitsuhiko Kimura, "Standards of Living in Colonial Korea: Did the Masses Become Worse Off or Better Off under Japanese Rule?" *Journal of Economic History* 53 (1993): 629–52; and Michael J. Seth, *Education Fever: Society, Politics, and the Pursuit of Schooling in South Korea* (Honolulu: University of Hawaii Press, 2002), pp. 9–33.

41. H.-Y. Lee, "Demographic Transition in Korea," pp. 5–17.

42. Paul W. Kuznets, *Korean Economic Development: An Interpretive Model* (Westport, CT: Praeger, 1994), pp. 25–28.

43. T.-H. Kim, *Mortality Transition,* p. 7; and Tai-Hwan Kwon, Hae Young Lee, Yun Shik Chung, and Eui-Young Yu, *The Population of Korea* (Seoul: Population and Development Studies Center, Seoul National University, 1975), pp. 19–23. Kwon and Kim, "Population of Korea," pp. 157–59, report that tuberculosis remained the third or fourth leading cause of death in the period 1958–62, having been the fourth leading cause during 1938–42.

44. Japanese owners had held 63 percent of cultivated land and 94 percent of manufacturing facilities. Chung H. Lee, *The Economic Transformation of South Korea: Lessons for the Transition Economies* (Paris: Development Center of the Organization for Economic Cooperation and Development, 1995), pp. 9 and 20.

45. Irma Adelman, "Social Development in Korea, 1953–1993," unpublished paper dated 1995, available as of December 12, 2004, at http://are.berkeley.edu/~adelman/KOREA.html; and Yoong-Deok Jeon and Young-Yong Kim, "Land Reform, Income Redistribution, and Agricultural Production in Korea," *Economic Development and Cultural Change* 48 (2000): 253–68. Urbanization may also have contributed to income equality.

46. Joseph A. Martellaro, "South Korea and Taiwan: A Comparative Analysis of the Generation and Distribution of Income," *Revista internazionale de scienza economiche e commerciali* 36 (1989): 1123–40; and UNDP World Income Inequality Database, accessed December 2, 2004.

47. Jong-Il You, "Income Distribution and Growth in East Asia," *Journal of Development Studies* 34 (1998): 37–65.

48. Adelman, "Social Development"; and Seth, *Education Fever,* p. 5. Noel F. McGinn et al., *Education and Development in Korea* (Cambridge, MA: Council on East Asian Studies, Harvard University, 1980), argue that education did not produce economic growth, but do not address health issues.

49. Adelman, "Social Development."

50. T.-H. Kwon, *Trends and Patterns of Mortality.*

4. Very Low Income Is Not a Barrier

1. Meegama traces the beginning of gains in life expectancy to the late nineteenth century. S. A. Meegama, "Cholera Epidemics and Their Control in Ceylon," *Population Studies* 33 (1979): 143–56; and Meegama, "The Decline of Mortality in Sri Lanka in Historical Perspective," *International Population Conference Manila 1981,* 3 vols. (Liège: International Union for the Scientific Study of Population, 1981), 2: 143–64. Sarkar prefers the early 1900s, and Roche the beginning of the 1900s. N. K. Sarkar, *The Demography of Ceylon* (Colombo: Ceylon Government Press, 1957); and Frederick C. Roche, "The Demographic Transition in Sri Lanka: Is Development Really a Prerequisite?," unpublished paper, Cornell University, 1976. Ramachandran selects 1923, and Gunatilleke points to the 1930s. P. Ramachandran, *Mortality Trends in Ceylon and the Federation of Malaysia* (Bombay: Demographic Training and Research Center, 1959); Godfrey Gunatilleke, "Health and Development in Sri Lanka—An Overview," in *Good Health at Low Cost,* ed. Scott B. Halstead, Julia A. Walsh, and Kenneth S. Warren (New York: Rockefeller Foundation, 1985), pp. 111–24. A United Nations source and Langford and Storey locate the beginning "after 1921" but in the 1920s, which is the interpretation accepted here. United Nations, Economic and Social Commission for Asia and the Pacific, *Population of Sri Lanka* (Bangkok: Economic and Social Commission for Asia and the Pacific, 1976); and Christopher Langford and Pamela Storey, "Sex Differentials in Mortality Early in the Twentieth Century: Sri Lanka and India Compared," *Population and Development Review* 19 (1993): 263–82.

2. United Nations, *Population of Sri Lanka,* p. 125.

3. But because underreporting of deaths persisted into the 1960s, these estimates may be slightly too high through those years.

4. James C. Riley, "Bibliography of Works Providing Estimates of Life Expectancy at Birth and of the Beginning Period of Health Transitions in Countries with a Population in 2000 of at least 400,000" at www.lifetable.de/RileyBib.htm, with comments on sources preferred for certain estimates.

5. On the epidemic see Margaret Jones, "The Ceylon Malaria Epidemic of 1934–35: A Case Study in Colonial Medicine," *Social History of Medicine* 13 (2000): 87–109.

6. Infant mortality dropped from 19.3 deaths per 1,000 live births in 1990 to 11.2 in 2002 and 2003, with more rapid gains occurring after 1997. Sri Lanka, Department of Census and Statistics, *Statistical Pocket Book of the Democratic Social-*

ist Republic of Sri Lanka (Colombo: Department of Census and Statistics, 2004), table 2.14.

7. Lloyd G. Reynolds, *Economic Growth in the Third World, 1850–1980* (New Haven: Yale University Press, 1985), pp. 136–38, describes the period 1880–1950 as an era of "intensive" economic growth.

8. While some sources regard this campaign as a great success (see United Nations, *Population of Sri Lanka,* p. 127; and C. G. Uragoda, "Rockefeller Philanthropy in the Development of Public Health in Sri Lanka," in *Philanthropy and Cultural Context: Western Philanthropy in South, East, and Southeast Asia in the Twentieth* ed. Soma Hewa and Philo Hove [Lanham, MD: University Press of America, 1997], pp. 65–81), others express reservations about its successes on plantations, though not in village households (see Soma Hewa, "The Hookworm Epidemic on the Plantations in Colonial Sri Lanka," *Medical History* 38 [1994]: 73–90; and Hewa, *Colonialism, Tropical Disease and Imperial Medicine: Rockefeller Philanthropy in Sri Lanka* [Lanham, MD: University Press of America, 1995]).

Commentators in the 1920s associated hookworm infection and its sequel anemia with tuberculosis and higher tuberculosis mortality. This has been substantiated by modern research. See Gadi Borkow and Zvi Bentwich, "Geohelminths, HIV/AIDS and TB," in *The Geohelminths: Ascaris, Trichuris, and Hookworm,* ed. Celia V. Holland and Malcolm W. Kennedy (Boston, 2001), pp. 301–17. Hookworm surveys in the late 1940s showed that infection levels remained low, which indicates that latrines continued to be used.

9. Margaret Jones, "Infant and Maternal Health Services in Ceylon, 1900–1948: Imperialism or Welfare?" *Social History of Medicine* 15 (2002): 263–90; and see Hewa, *Colonialism, Tropical Disease and Imperial Medicine.*

10. Patricia Alailama and Nimal Sanderatne, "Social Policies in a Slow Growth Economy: Sri Lanka," in *Development with a Human Face: Experiences in Social Achievement and Economic Growth,* ed. Santosh Mehrotra and Richard Jolly (Oxford: Clarendon Press, 1997), pp. 235–63. Gunatilleke, "Health and Development in Sri Lanka"; and Roche, *Demographic Transition in Sri Lanka.*

11. James Warner Björkman, "Health Policy and Politics in Sri Lanka: Developments in the South Asian Welfare State," *Asian Survey* 25 (1985): 537–52.

12. E.g., H. R. Seneviratne and L. C. Rajapaksa, "Safe Motherhood in Sri Lanka: A 100-Year March," *International Journal of Gynecology and Obstetrics* 70 (2000): 113–24; and E. L. Wijemanne, "Population Growth and Educational Development," in United Nations, *Population of Sri Lanka,* pp. 208–33.

13. Anju Malhotra and Deborah S. DeGraff, "Daughters and Wives: Marital Status, Poverty, and Young Women's Employment in Sri Lanka," in *Women, Poverty, and Demographic Change,* ed. Brígida García (Oxford: Oxford University Press, 2000), pp. 145–74, report that the position of females in Sri Lanka had historically been favorable, but figure 15 makes evident the limits to that generalization in schooling and literacy. So, too, do the literacy rates reported by Björkman ("Health Policy and Politics," p. 545), from 1881 to 1981, which show that female literacy lagged male literacy throughout. And see Lakshman Dissanayake, "The Timing and Determinants of the Onset of Mass Education in Sri Lanka," *Asian*

Profile 23 (1995): 223–34, on the rising proportion of school-age children attending school.

14. Sources arguing for major DDT-related decline are A. N. A. Abeyesundere, "Recent Trends in Malaria Morbidity and Mortality in Sri Lanka," in *Population Problems of Sri Lanka*, ed. G. Abayasekera (Colombo: Demographic Training and Research Unit, University of Sri Lanka, 1976), pp. 48–66; O. E. R. Abhayaratne, "The Influence of Malaria on Infant Mortality in Ceylon," *Ceylon Journal of Medical Science* 7 (1950): 33–54; H. Cullumbine, "An Analysis of the Vital Statistics of Ceylon," *Ceylon Journal of Medical Science* 7 (1950): 133–42; R. H. Gray, "The Decline of Mortality in Ceylon and the Demographic Effects of Malaria Control," *Population Studies* 28 (1974): 205–29; P. R. Newman, *Malaria Eradication and Population Growth with Special Reference to Ceylon and British Guiana* (Ann Arbor: School of Public Health, University of Michigan, 1965); and Jayaratne Pinikahana and Robert A. Dixon, "Trends in Malaria Morbidity and Mortality in Sri Lanka," *Journal of Malariology* 30 (1993): 51–55. Others express doubts: H. Frederiksen, "Malaria Eradication and the Fall of Mortality," *Population Studies* 24 (1970): 111–13; Christopher Langford, "Reasons for the Decline in Mortality in Sri Lanka Immediately after the Second World War: A Re-examination of the Evidence," *Health Transition Review* 6 (1996): 3–23; S. A. Meegama, "Malaria Eradication and Its Effect on Mortality Levels," *Population Studies* 21 (1967): 207–37; and Sarkar, *Demography of Ceylon*.

15. Abeyesundere, "Recent Trends," pp. 60–61.

16. Bruce Caldwell, "The Family and Demographic Change in Sri Lanka," *Health Transition Review*, Supplement, 6 (1996): 45–60, reports on a 1985–87 survey that included a series of questions on mortality posed to older women. Respondents cited better health facilities provided by the government, better understanding among parents about health risks, and behavioral changes as factors in improved survival.

17. Seneviratne and Rajapaksa, "Safe Motherhood."

18. Meegama, "Decline of Mortality in Sri Lanka," 2: 143–64; and Srinivasa A. Meegama, "Obstacles to the Further Decline of Mortality in Sri Lanka—The Experience of the Last Two Decades," in *Mortality in South and East Asia: A Review of Changing Trends and Patterns, 1950–1975* (Manila: World Health Organization, 1982), pp. 355–76.

19. Dallas F. S. Fernando, "Health Statistics in Sri Lanka, 1921–80," in *Good Health at Low Cost*, ed. Scott B. Halstead, Julia A. Walsh, and Kenneth S. Warren (New York: Rockefeller Foundation, 1985), pp. 79–92.

20. Godfrey Gunatilleke, "Sri Lanka's Social Achievements and Challenges," in *Social Development and Public Policy: A Study of Some Successful Experiences*, ed. Dharam Ghai (New York: St. Martin's Press, 2000), p. 140 for the quote and pp. 164–78. On continuing poor nutrition into the 1990s, see H. R. Gunasekera, *Nutrition Status of Children in Sri Lanka: Findings from Demographic and Health Surveys* (Colombo: Department of Census and Statistics, 1996); and World Bank, *Attaining the Millennium Development Goals in Sri Lanka: How Likely and What Will It Take to Reduce Poverty, Child Mortality and Malnutrition, and to Increase*

School Enrollment and Completion? February, 2005, available online at siteresources. worldbank.org/INTSRILANKA/Resources/Sri-Lanka-MDG-Final.pdf, accessed May 25, 2006.

5. Two Neighbors

1. The most thorough description of these techniques is given by Joseph A. Le Prince and A. J. Orenstein, *Mosquito Control in Panama: The Eradication of Malaria and Yellow Fever in Cuba and Panama* (New York: Putnam, 1916). The Gorgas method was used in Havana, in the Canal Zone in Panama, and in Japan in the early years of U.S. occupation after World War II.

2. The British West Indies supplied some 60 percent of all employees, mostly black laborers. See Velma Newton, *The Silver Men: West Indian Labour Migration to Panama, 1850–1914,* rev. ed. (Kingston, Jamaica: Ian Randle, 2004), esp. pp. 46, 88–94, 154.

3. Weston P. Chamberlain, *Twenty-five Years of American Medical Activity on the Isthmus of Panama, 1904–1929: A Triumph of Preventive Medicine* (Mount Hope, Canal Zone: Panama Canal Press, 1929), esp. pp. 12–17, 29–35; and J. P. McLaren, *A Brief History of Sanitation in the Canal Zone, 1513–1972: Environmental Health* (n.p.: n.p., 1972), esp. pp. 10–24. See also David Ray Abernathy, "Bound to Succeed: Science, Territoriality, and the Emergence of Disease Eradication in the Panama Canal Zone" (PhD diss., University of Washington, 2000).

4. "In a large part of this country the incidence of the disease [malaria] is probably as high as it ever was," according to James Stevens Simmons et al., *Malaria in Panama* (Baltimore: Johns Hopkins Press, 1939), p. 56, writing about the results of surveys in many regions.

5. James K. Fowler, *An Impression of Jamaica and the Panama Canal Zone* (London: Eyre and Spottiswoode, 1924), pp. 47–49, quote from p. 47. Fowler hoped (pp. 53–54) for some way to control mosquitoes outside the two-mile band in order to protect the crews of ships using the canal!

6. John Biesanz and Mavis Biesanz, *The People of Panama* (New York: Columbia University Press, 1955), e.g., pp. 254–55. The Biesanzes detected very recent improvements in tuberculosis mortality, however.

7. United States Bureau of the Census, *Panama: Summary of Biostatistics* (Washington: Bureau of the Census, 1945), pp. 57 and 67, reports that official records on mortality and infant mortality were defective.

8. Omar Jaén Suárez, *La población del Istmo de Panamá: Estudio de geohistoria,* 3rd ed. (Madrid: Ediciónes de Cultura Hispánica, 1998), pp. 114, 497; and Robert E. Looney, *The Economic Development of Panama: The Impact of World Inflation on an Open Economy* (New York: Praeger, 1976), pp. 1, 7–8, 37, 40, and 42–45. Gloria Rudolf, *Panama's Poor: Victims, Agents, and Historymakers* (Gainesville: University Press of Florida, 1999), pp. 62–80, argues that conditions in rural areas deteriorated between the 1920s and 1960s, especially in work opportunities and diets. On the period after 1968, and especially on the 1990s, see Carlos Correa,

Enoch Adames, and Raúl Leis, *Gobernabilidad democrática y seguridad ciudadana en Centroamérica: El caso de Panamá* (Managua: CRIES, 2001).

9. Héctor Pérez Brignoli, "Notas sobre el descenso de la mortalidad en Costa Rica (1866–1973)," in *Sétimo seminario nacional de demografía* (San José: n.p., 1979), pp. 44–56; and Pérez Brignoli, *El crecimiento demográfico de America Latina en los siglos XIX y XX: Problemas, metodos y perspectives* (San Jose: Centro de Investigaciónes Historicas, Universidad de Costa Rica, 1989), p. 12. And Luis Rosero Bixby, "Determinantes del descenso de la mortalidad infantil en Costa Rica," in *Demografía y epidemiología en Costa Rica* (San José: Asociación Demográfica Costarricense, 1985), pp. 9–36; Leonardo Mata and Rosero Bixby, *National Health and Social Development in Costa Rica: A Case Study of Intersectoral Action* (Washington: Pan American Health Organization, 1988); and Rosero Bixby and Herman Caamaño, "Tablas de vida de Costa Rica, 1900–1980," in *Mortalidad y fecundidad en Costa Rica* (San José: Asociación Demográfica Costarricense, 1984), pp. 7–19.

10. Mario Samper, *Generations of Settlers: Rural Households and Markets on the Costa Rican Frontier, 1850–1935* (Boulder, CO: Westview Press, 1990), pp. 119–20, also sees the latter part of the nineteenth century as a period of gains in survival.

11. On Jamaicans and others in Costa Rica, see Aviva Chomsky, *West Indian Workers and the United Fruit Company in Costa Rica, 1870–1940* (Baton Rouge: Louisiana State University Press, 1996), esp. pp. 89–103.

12. Astrid Fischel, "Politics and Education in Costa Rica, 1880–1930" (PhD diss., University of Southampton, 1991), p. 45; Mata and Rosero Bixby, *National Health and Social Development in Costa Rica;* Stacy May et al., *Costa Rica: A Study in Economic Development* (New York: Twentieth-Century Fund, 1952), p. 102; Carmelo Mesa-Lago, *Market, Socialism and Mixed Economies: Comparative Policy and Performance, Chile, Cuba, and Costa Rica* (Baltimore: Johns Hopkins University Press, 2000), esp. pp. 402–11; Steven Palmer and Gladys Rojas Chaves, "Educating Señorita: Teacher Training, Social Mobility, and the Birth of Costa Rican Feminism, 1885–1925," *Hispanic American Historical Review* 78 (1998): 45–82; Pérez Brignoli, "Notas sobre el descenso de la mortalidad en Costa Rica," pp. 44–56; Luis Rosero Bixby, "Socioeconomic Development, Health Interventions and Mortality Decline in Costa Rica," *Scandinavian Journal of Social Medicine* 46, supplement (1990): 33–42; and Juan Diego Trajos, "Costa Rica: The State's Response to Poverty," in *Strategies to Combat Poverty in Latin America,* ed. Dagmar Raczynski (Washington: Inter-American Development Bank, 1995), pp. 149–205

13. Ana Cecilia Román Trigo, *Las finanzas públicas de Costa Rica: Metodología y fuentes (1870–1948)* (San José: Centro de Investigaciónes Históricas de América Central, Universidad de Costa Rica, 1995), pp. 56–63.

14. Chomsky, *West Indian Workers,* pp. 100–11 and 132–33. Initial reports on the use of the synthetic quinine-substitute Plasmochin (also called plasmoquin or plasmoquine) in Costa Rica were promising, but further testing produced mixed results. J. W. Field et al., "Field Observations on the Effects of Prophylactic Plasmoquine on the Incidence, Course, Severity and Transmission of P. vivax Malaria," *Bulletin from the Institute for Medical Research, Federated Malay*

States No. 3 (1940), concluded that plasmoquine had little or no effect in their field test.

15. Mata and Rosero, *National Health and Social Development,* quote from p. 59. Juliana Martínez, "Policy Environments and Selective Emulation in the Making of Health Policies: The Case of Costa Rica, 1920–1997" (PhD diss., University of Pittsburgh, 1998), argues that Costa Rican elites selectively adopted ideas and policies about health from abroad beginning in the period 1920–48, and that this approach explains why the country achieved high life expectancy; see her pp. 44–78 on the period 1920–48.

16. E.g., Claudio González-Vega and Víctor Hugo Céspedes, "Costa Rica," in *Costa Rica and Uruguay,* ed. Simon Rottenberg (Washington: World Bank, 1993), pp. 59–74.

17. Ibid., pp. 43–58. I have been unable to uncover information about income distribution between the 1890s and the 1950s. On the more recent period see especially Samuel A. Morley, *Poverty and Inequality in Latin America: The Impact of Adjustment and Recovery in the 1980s* (Baltimore: Johns Hopkins University Press, 1995), p. 30. The different estimates given by Morley for the period 1979–88 show an average Gini coefficient of 40.3.

18. Chomsky, *West Indian Workers,* pp. 101–3; Leonardo Mata, "The Fight against Diarrheal Diseases: The Case of Costa Rica," in *Health Policy, Social Policy and Mortality Prospects,* ed. Jacques Vallin and Alan D. Lopez (Liège: Ordina Editions, 1985), pp. 57–79; Mata and Rosero, *National Health and Social Development;* May et al., *Costa Rica,* esp. pp. 187–89, 196–99; Edgard Mohs, *La salud en Costa Rica* (San José: Editorial Universidad Estatal a Distancia, 1983), esp. pp. 37–59; Iván Molina Jiménez, "Clase, género y etnia van a la escuela: El Alfabetismo en Costa Rica y Nicaragua (1880–1950)," in *Educando a Costa Rica: Alfabetización popular, formación docente y género (1880–1950),* ed. Iván Molina and Steven Palmer (San José: Editorial Porvenir, 2000), p. 34; Pérez Brignoli, "Notas sobre el descenso de la mortalidad en Costa Rica"; and Luis Rosero Bixby, "Infant Mortality Decline in Costa Rica," in *Good Health at Low Cost,* ed. Scott B. Halstead, Julia A. Walsh, and Kenneth S. Warren (New York: Rockefeller Foundation, 1985), pp. 125–58. Some commentators, e.g. Claudio Gonzalez-Vega, "Health Improvements in Costa Rica: The Socioeconomic Background," in *Good Health at Low Cost,* pp. 147–58, stress factors associated with the 1960s and 1970s even while acknowledging that gains began earlier.

On the hookworm campaign, see Steven Palmer, *From Popular Medicine to Medical Populism: Doctors, Healers, and Public Power in Costa Rica, 1800–1940* (Durham, NC: Duke University Press, 2003), pp. 155–82; and Palmer, "El Mago de Coney Island Park," in *La Voluntad radiante: Culture impresa, magia y medicina en Costa Rica (1897–1932),* ed. Iván Molina Jiménez and Steven Palmer (San José: Editorial Porvenir, 1996), pp. 111–15.

19. Palmer, "El Mago de Coney Island Park," pp. 111–20.

20. On the 1960s and 1970s see esp. Ludwig Gündel G. and Juan Diego Trejos S., *Reformas recientes en el sector salud de Costa Rica* (Santiago de Chile: United Nations, Economic Commission for Latin America and the Caribbean, 1994), pp.

11–15. And see Setha M. Low, *Culture, Politics and Medicine in Costa Rica: An Anthropological Study of Medical Change* (Bedford Hills, NY: Redgrave Publishing Co., 1985); Carmelo Mesa-Lago, "Health Care in Costa Rica: Boom and Crisis," *Social Science and Medicine* 21 (1985): 13–21; and Lynn M. Morgan, "Health without Wealth? Costa Rica's Health System under Economic Crisis," *Journal of Public Health Policy* 8 (1987): 86–105. José F. Betancourt, "Different Roads to a Common Goal: The Lowering of Infant Mortality Rates in Latin America," *Revista Geografica* 107 (1988): 49–66, maintains that female autonomy played a role in reducing infant mortality.

James W. McGuire, "Social Policy and Mortality Decline in East Asia and Latin America," *World Development* 29 (2001): 1673–97, argues that health policies initiated in the 1960s and 1970s allowed Costa Rica to keep up with Taiwan and South Korea in reducing infant mortality. But William H. Dow and Kammi K. Schmeer, "Health Insurance and Child Mortality in Costa Rica," *Social Science and Medicine* 57 (2003): 975–86, test and find little support for the hypothesis that expanded coverage in the 1970s led to lower child mortality. Chomsky, *West Indian Workers,* pp. 93–94 reports that the United Fruit Company funded its program of medical services for employees by deducting 2 percent from wages.

6. Capitalism and Communism, Dictatorship and Democracy

1. Life expectancy in Cuba varied sharply from period to period during 1865 to 1900, dropping to a critically low level during the Spanish-American War of 1898. From about 1900 to 1960 authorities differ in their estimates, with the discrepancy peaking in the 1920s at three or four years. The estimate for Jamaica around 1830 refers to the slave population of the British West Indies; slaves then dominated in Jamaica's population.

2. Rolando Garcia Quiñones, *La transition de la mortalidad en Cuba: Un estudio sociodemográfico* (Havana: Centro de Estudios Demográficos, Universidad de la Habana, 1996), pp. 48, 87–8, 102, and annex; and Alfonso Farnós Morejón, "Los niveles de mortalidad en Cuba durante el siglo XX," *Revista cubana de administración de salud* 3 (1977): 351–63, citing Elio Velázquez and Lázaro Toirac, *Cuba: Tablas de mortalidad estimadas por sexo, para los años calendario terminados en cero y cinco durante el periodo 1900–1950* (Havana: Centro de Estudio Demográficos, Universidad de la Habana, 1975).

3. James C. Riley, *Poverty and Life Expectancy: The Jamaica Paradox* (Cambridge: Cambridge University Press, 2005), pp. 26–27.

4. Dudley Seers et al., *Cuba: The Economic and Social Revolution* (Chapel Hill: University of North Carolina Press, 1964), p. 7. That would mean, using Angus Maddison's estimates of U.S. GDPpc in the same years (*The World Economy: Historical Statistics* [Paris: Development Center of the Organization for Economic

Cooperation and Development, 2003], p. 88), a Cuban GDPpc of more than I$ 2,119.

5. Alejandro de la Fuente, *A Nation for All: Race, Inequality, and Politics in Twentieth-Century Cuba* (Chapel Hill: University of North Carolina Press, 2001), pp. 95 and 115–17.

6. Sergio Diaz-Briquets, *The Health Revolution in Cuba* (Austin: University of Texas Press, 1983), esp. pp. 28–51; Garcia Quiñones, *La transition de la mortalidad en Cuba,* pp. 19–49 and 87–109; and James W. McGuire and Laura B. Frankel, "Mortality Decline in Cuba, 1900–1959: Patterns, Comparisons, and Causes," *Latin American Research Review* 40 (2005): 83–116.

7. José A. López del Valle, *The Development of Sanitation and Charities in Cuba during the Last Sixteen Years (1899–1914)* (Havana: La Moderna Poesía, 1914).

8. Diaz-Briquets, *The Health Revolution in Cuba,* esp. pp. 67–101.

9. Thus the 1953 census showed that about the same proportion of people in the age ranges 20–24 up to 50–54 had attended primary school. On education see the section by Richard Jolly in Seers et al., *Cuba: The Economic and Social Revolution,* pp. 166–69.

10. De la Fuente, *A Nation for All,* pp. 139–47.

11. Aviva Chomsky, "'The Threat of a Good Example': Health and Revolution in Cuba," in *Dying for Growth: Global Inequality and the Health of the Poor,* ed. Jim Yong Kim (Monroe, ME: Common Courage Press, 2000), pp. 331–58; Diaz-Briquets, *Health Revolution in Cuba;* Hector Gutiérrez, "La mortalité par cause à Cuba, avant et après la Révolution," *Population* 39 (1984): 383–88; Raúl Hernández Castellon, *Le Revolución demográfica en Cuba* (Havana: Editorial de Ciencias Sociales, 1988); Theodore MacDonald, *Making a New People: Education in Revolutionary Cuba* (Vancouver: New Star Books, 1985); Raúl L. Riverón Corteguera, "Strategies and Causes of Reduced Infant and Young Child Diarrheal Disease Mortality in Cuba, 1962–1993," *Bulletin of the PAHO* 29 (1995): 70–80; and Howard Waitzkin, *The Politics of Medical Encounters: How Patients and Doctors Deal with Social Problems* (New Haven: Yale University Press, 1991).

For a critique of the postrevolutionary health system see David Werner, "Health Care in Cuba: A Model Service or a Means of Social Control—or Both?" in *Practising Health for All,* ed. David Morley, Jon E. Rohde, and Glen Williams (Oxford: Oxford University Press, 1983), pp. 17–37. On effects of the U.S. embargo, see Richard Garfield and Sarah Santana, "The Impact of the Economic Crisis and the U.S. Embargo on Health in Cuba," *American Journal of Public Health* 87 (1997): 15–20. On Cuban medical aid to developing countries, see Julie Margot Feinsilver, *Healing the Masses: Cuban Health Politics at Home and Abroad* (Berkeley: University of California Press, 1993). On the 1990s, see Carmelo Mesa-Lago, "Assessing Economic and Social Performance in the Cuban Transition of the 1990s," *World Development* 26 (1998): 857–76. And for an assessment of Cuba's postrevolutionary emphasis on social over economic development, see Elena Álvarez and Jorge Máttar, eds., *Política social y reformas estructurales: Cuba a principios del siglo XXI* (Mexico City: Comisión Económica para América Latina y el Caribe, 2004).

12. Cuba also began sending physicians and medical missions abroad, ultimately to some sixty countries. Feinsilver, *Healing the Masses.*

13. De la Fuente, *A Nation for All,* p. 309; and Alejandro de la Fuente, "Race and Inequality in Cuba, 1899–1981," *Journal of Contemporary History* 30 (1995): 131–68.

14. On the most recent period especially see Jerry M. Spiegel and Annalee Yassi, "Lessons from the Margins of Globalization: Appreciating the Cuban Health Paradox," *Journal of Public Health Policy* 25 (2004): 85–110.

15. This section draws on Riley, *Poverty and Life Expectancy,* esp. pp. 52–58.

7. The Soviet and Chinese Models of Social Development

1. The term "communist" distinguishes economic and social policies followed by the Soviet Union and China from "socialist" policies followed by the West European social democracies, Costa Rica, Sri Lanka, and Kerala state in India.

2. Thus Ethiopia and Tanzania are excluded for having followed the model too briefly, although perhaps also without the requisite resources or political authority.

3. Up to 1989 estimates for Ukraine are also incorporated in estimates for the Soviet Union.

4. Alain Blum, *Naître, vivre et mourir en URSS, 1917–1991* (Paris: A. Michel, 1994), pp. 146 and 149, reading from charts; and Blum, "De la population soviétique à la population russe: Un destin atypique," in *La population du monde: Enjeux et problèmes,* ed. Jean-Claude Chasteland and Jean-Claude Chesnais (Paris: Presses universitaires de France, 1997), p. 316.

5. Natalia Ksenofontova, "Trends in Infant Mortality in the USSR," in *Demographic Trends and Patterns in the Soviet Union before 1991,* ed. Wolfgang Lutz, Sergei Scherbov, and Andrei Volkov (London: Routledge, 1994), pp. 359–78.

6. France Meslé and Jacques Vallin, *Mortalité et causes de décès en Ukraine au XXe siècle* (Paris: Institut national d'études démographiques, 2003); S. A. Tomiline, *Organisation d'hygiène: L'hygiène publique dans la population rurale de l'Ukraine* ([Chambéry]: n.p., 1925); and Jacques Vallin et al., "A New Estimate of Ukrainian Population Losses during the Crises of the 1930s and 1940s," *Population Studies* 56 (2002): 249–64.

7. However, Leonard Jan Bruce-Chwatt and Julian de Zulueta, *The Rise and Fall of Malaria in Europe: A Historico-Epidemiological Study* (Oxford: Oxford University Press, 1980), p. 29, report one successful project in the 1930s in the salinification of a brackish marsh, thus reducing breeding opportunities for anopheles mosquitoes.

8. Arjan Gjonça, *Communism, Health and Lifestyle: The Paradox of Mortality Transition in Albania, 1950–1990* (Westport, CT: Greenwood Press, 2001), esp. pp. 15–35; and Ermelinda Meksi and Gianpiero Dalla Zuanna, "La mortalité générale

en Albanie (1950–1990)," *Population* 49 (1994): 607–36. Gjonça argues that Albania's Mediterranean diet and lifestyle contributed to life expectancy, presumably meaning to underlying advantages and a comparatively high initial level. Kirsten D. Senturia, "Maternal and Child Health in Albania," *Social Science and Medicine* 43 (1996): 1097–1107, reports results of a 1993–94 survey, the aim of which was to determine whether female and infant health were actually as good as reported. She found that they were, despite the deterioration of health services in recent years. Vefik Qerimi, *Public Health Service in the People's Republic of Albania* (Tirana: Naim Frashëri, 1967), gives some information about malaria control and about the meager health system of the 1930s.

9. Anthony Clunies-Ross and Petar Sudar, eds., *Albania's Economy in Transition and Turmoil, 1990–97* (Brookfield, VT: Ashgate Pub., 1998), esp. pp. 35–36 and 162.

10. For a discussion of the various estimates, see John Caldwell et al., "Population Trends in China—A Perspective Provided by the 1982 Census," in *A Census of One Billion People,* ed. Chengrui Li (Hong Kong: Economic Information and Agency, 1986), pp. 352–91; and James Lee and Wang Feng, *One Quarter of Humanity: Malthusian Mythology and Chinese Realities, 1700–2000* (Cambridge, MA: Harvard University Press, 1999), pp. 54–55. Janet W. Salaff, "Mortality Decline in the People's Republic of China and the United States," *Population Studies* 27 (1973): 551–76, adds estimates of crude death rates from Chinese sources.

11. F. P. Lisowski, "The Emergence and Development of the Barefoot Doctor in China," *Eastern Horizon* 19 (1980): 7; and R. M. Worth, "Rural Health in China: From Village to Commune," *American Journal of Hygiene* 77 (1963): 228–39.

12. On economic gains in the 1920s and 1930s, see Marie-Claire Bergère, *The Golden Age of the Chinese Bourgeoisie, 1911–1937* (Cambridge: Cambridge University Press, 1989), esp. pp. 63–77; and Thomas G. Rawski, *Economic Growth in Prewar China* (Berkeley: University of California Press, 1989), p. 341. On public sector spending on health and education see Arthur N. Young, *China's Nation-Building Effort, 1927–1937: The Financial and Economic Record* (Stanford, CA: Hoover Institution Press, 1971), pp. 77–79 and 359.

13. On life expectancy in China, in addition to the sources cited below, see Sheng Luo, "Reconstruction of Life Tables and Age Distributions for the Population of China, by Year, from 1953 to 1982" (PhD diss., University of Pennsylvania, 1988), pp. 150–65; Hao Hong Sheng, "Mortality Levels, Trends and Differentials in China," in *Differential Development and Demographic Dilemma: Perspectives from China and India,* ed. Kuttan Mahadevan et al. (Delhi: B. R. Publishing Co, 1994), pp. 225–49; and Rui Yan and Shengli Chen, "A Study of the Mortality Rate and Life Expectancy of the Chinese Population over the Last Forty Years," *Chinese Journal of Population Science* 3 (1991): 259–75.

14. On the decline in life expectancy in the recent period, see Elizabeth Brainerd and David M. Cutler, "Autopsy on an Empire: Understanding Mortality in Russia and the Former Soviet Union," *Journal of Economic Perspectives* 19 (2005): 107–30.

15. Meslé and Vallin, *Mortalité et causes de décès,* pp. 250–63. World Bank, *Dying Too Young: Addressing Premature Mortality and Ill Health Due to Non-Com-*

municable Diseases and Injuries in the Russian Federation (Washington: World Bank, 2005), assesses effects of these causes of death on life expectancy (accessed June 6, 2006, at siteresources.worldbank.org/INTECA/Resources/DTY-Final.pdf).

16. William A. Knaus, *Inside Russian Medicine: An American Doctor's First-Hand Report* (Boston: Everest House, 1981), p. 13; the quoted comment is from Urii Lisitsin.

17. Richard Johnson, "Malaria and Malaria Control in the USSR, 1917–1941" (PhD diss., Georgetown University, 1988).

18. W. Horsley Gantt, *A Medical Review of Soviet Russia* (London: British Medical Association, 1928), pp. 41–51; and S. G. Wheatcroft, "Population Dynamic and Factors Affecting It, in the Soviet Union in the 1920s and 1930s," unpublished typescript, 1976, p. 107 (Wheatcroft discusses malaria on pp. 110–22).

19. E. Thomas Ewing, *The Teachers of Stalinism: Policy, Practice, and Power in Soviet Schools of the 1930s* (New York: P. Lang, 2002), p. 5. Ben Eklof, *Russian Peasant Schools: Officialdom, Village Culture, and Popular Pedagogy, 1864–1914* (Berkeley: University of California Press, 1986), pp. 187 and 285, reports that 44–46 percent of children aged 8–11 were enrolled in schools in 1911, though many fewer girls than boys.

20. David M. Heer, "The Demographic Transition in the Russian Empire and the Soviet Union," *Journal of Social History* (1968): 193–240; see p. 223. Selecting the age group 9–49 of course biases these rates upward.

21. Ewing, *Teachers of Stalinism,* p. 5.

22. Ibid., esp. pp. 57–68.

23. Sheila Fitzpatrick, *Education and Social Mobility in the Soviet Union, 1921–1934* (Cambridge: Cambridge University Press, 1979), esp. pp. 159–76; and, on the 1931 reform, Larry E. Holmes, *Stalin's School: Moscow's Model School No. 25, 1931–1937* (Pittsburgh: University of Pittsburgh Press, 1999), pp. 10–12.

24. On the education system in the 1950s and 1960s see Mervyn Matthews, *Education in the Soviet Union: Policies and Institutions since Stalin* (London: Allen & Unwin, 1982).

25. On the zemstvo effort and its shortcomings, see Robert Philippot, *Société civile et état bureaucratique dans la Russie tsariste: Les zemstvos* (Paris: Institut d'études slaves, 1991), esp. pp. 87–96. Also Samuel C. Ramer, "Feldshers and Rural Health Care in the Early Soviet Period," in *Health and Society in Revolutionary Russia,* ed. Susan Gross Solomon and John F. Hutchinson (Bloomington: Indiana University Press, 1990), pp. 121–45; and Henry E. Sigerist, *Medicine and Health in the Soviet Union* (New York: Citadel Press, 1947), pp. 10–21, 72–73, and 251.

26. Heer, "Demographic Transition in the Russian Empire," 222. Also, Sigerist, *Medicine and Health,* pp. 34–35, reports official estimates of numbers of medical facilities for 1913–41.

27. Knaus, *Inside Russian Medicine,* p. 88.

28. Lillian Li-ning Liu, "The Development of the Soviet Rural Health Care System and the Role of Feldshers, 1917–1941" (PhD diss., University of Maryland, 1988); and Sigerist, *Medicine and Health,* pp. 53–118.

29. Heinz Müller-Dietz, "Fifty Years of the Soviet Health Service," *Review of Soviet Medical Sciences* 6 (1969): 26–34.

30. Ramer, "Feldshers and Rural Health Care," pp. 121–45, quote from 134.

31. Knaus, *Inside Russian Medicine*, esp. p. 103 on shortages in medicines and equipment in the 1970s; and Michael Ryan, *Doctors and the State in the Soviet Union* (New York: St. Martin's Press, 1990), pp. 7 and 11–18 on medical training. Ryan also points out (pp. 19–25) that Soviet doctors were poorly paid by Soviet standards into the 1960s.

32. Gordon Hyde, *The Soviet Health Service: A Historical and Comparative Study* (London: Lawrence & Wishart, 1974), pp. 59–60. Landon Pearson, *Children of Glasnost: Growing Up Soviet* (Seattle: University of Washington Press, 1990), pp. 231–61, discusses ambitions for child health, going back to Lenin's ideals, and realities in the 1980s.

33. Christopher M. Davis, "Economics of Soviet Public Health, 1928–1932: Development Strategy, Resource Constraints, and Health Plans," in *Health and Society,* ed. Solomon and Hutchinson, p. 160.

34. Through the 1970s, equality in labor markets remained a goal not attained. See Alastair McAuley, *Women's Work and Wages in the Soviet Union* (London: Allen & Unwin, 1981).

35. See Norton T. Dodge, *Women in the Soviet Economy: Their Role in Economic, Scientific, and Technical Development* (Baltimore: Johns Hopkins Press, 1966). Dodge (p. 209) tracks the rising number and proportion of women physicians from 10 percent of the total in 1913 to 76 percent in 1950.

36. Madeleine Estryn-Behar and Abraham Behar, *Santé publique et médecine préventive en république populaire d'Albani*e ([Paris]: N. B. E., 1976), esp. pp. 34–40, provide details. Also Örjan Sjöberg, *Rural Change and Development in Albania* (Boulder, CO: Westview Press, 1991), esp. pp. 65–68 on schooling.

37. The most recent reworking of these estimates affirms rapid gains. Judith Banister and Kenneth Hill, "Mortality in China 1964–2000," *Population Studies* 58 (2004): 55–75.

38. Judith Banister, *China's Changing Population* (Stanford, CA: Stanford University Press, 1987), pp. 78–80, argues against the idea of survival gains in the 1920s or 1930s. But Cameron Campbell, "Public Health Efforts in China before 1949 and Their Effects on Mortality," *Social Science History* 21 (1997): 179–218, maintains that public health reforms in Beijing in the 1920s and 1930s reduced mortality. A number of authorities detail changes in public health and medicine in other parts of China in the 1920s and 1930s. See esp. C. C. Chen, *Medicine in Rural China: A Personal Account* (Berkeley: University of California Press, 1989), esp. pp. 17–20, who deals with hospital building, physician training, and efforts to educate the populace in disease prevention. Kerrie L. Macpherson, *A Wilderness of Marches: The Origins of Public Health in Shanghai, 1843–1893* (Hong Kong: Oxford University Press, 1987), pp. 44–45, argues that hygiene efforts improved health status without reducing mortality. In Tianjin effective steps to improve public health came only in the 1950s, but important foundations were laid during 1900–1902 by Japanese occupiers; see Ruth Rogaski, *Hygienic Modernity: Mean-*

ings of Health and Disease in Treaty-Port China (Berkeley: University of California Press, 2004).

39. Ka-che Yip, *Health and National Reconstruction in Nationalist China: The Development of Modern Health Services, 1928–1937* (Ann Arbor: Association for Asian Studies, 1995).

40. Conrad Seipp, ed., *Health Care for the Community: Selected Papers of John B. Grant* (Baltimore: Johns Hopkins Press, 1963), pp. 8–10 and 148–54; and Yip, *Health and National Reconstruction*.

41. Frederick C. Teiwes, "Establishment and Consolidation of the New Regime," in *The Cambridge History of China*, vol. 14, *The People's Republic*, part I: *The Emergence of Revolutionary China 1949–1965*, ed. Roderick MacFarquhar and John K. Fairbank (Cambridge: Cambridge University Press, 1987), pp. 57–58 and 63–67, discusses the wider context of following Soviet models in some areas but not in others. From 1958 onward a foreign policy dispute with the Soviet Union made Soviet models more problematic for the Chinese.

42. Carl E. Taylor, Robert L. Parker, and Zeng Dong-Lu, "Public Health Policies and Strategies in China," in *Oxford Textbook of Public Health*, ed. Walter W. Holland, Roger Detels, and George Knox, 2nd ed., 3 vols. (Oxford: Oxford University Press, 1991), 1: 261–69.

43. Worth, "Rural Health in China."

44. On individual toilet behaviors and composting, see esp. Andrew Morris, "'Fight for Fertilizer!': Excrement, Public Health, and Mobilization in New China," *Journal of Unconventional History* 6 (1995): 51–76.

45. Tao-Tai Hsia, "Laws on Public Health," in *Medicine and Public Health in the People's Republic of China*, ed. Joseph R. Quinn (Washington: National Institutes of Health, 1973), p. 114, gives a brief discussion of the 1940s efforts.

46. Peter Heller, "The Strategy of Health-Sector Planning," in *Public Health in the People's Republic of China: Report of a Conference*, ed. Myron E. Wegman, Tsung-yi Lin, and Elizabeth F. Purcell (New York: Josiah Macy Jr. Foundation, [1973]), pp. 62–107, quote from p. 72; and see Banister, *China's Changing Population*, esp. pp. 50–59, 78–85; S. M. Hillier and J. A. Jewell, *Health Care and Traditional Medicine in China, 1800–1982* (London: Routledge and Kegan Paul, 1983); Salaff, "Mortality Decline in the People's Republic of China"; and Xiao-Nong Zhou et al., "The Public Health Significance and Control of Schistosomiasis in China—Then and Now," *Acta Tropica* 96 (2005): 97–105. Dean T. Jamison et al., *China: The Health Sector* (Washington: World Bank, 1984), reports on the World Bank's 1982 survey of rural health.

47. Lisowski, "Emergence and Development," 9; Susan B. Rifkin, "Health Care for Rural Areas," in *Medicine and Public Health in the People's Republic of China*, ed. Joseph R. Quinn (Washington: National Institutes of Health, 1973), pp. 141–52; and Victor Sidel, "Medical Personnel and Their Training," in *Medicine and Public Health*, pp. 153–72. Hygiene workers were trained for six months, and auxiliary medical workers for two years. About 80 percent of China's population lived in rural areas in the 1950s.

48. Mary Brown Bullock, *An American Transplant: The Rockefeller Foundation*

and Peking Medical College (Berkeley: University of California Press, 1980), pp. 162–89; and Taylor, et al., "Public Health Policies," 261–69.

49. Sidel, "Medical Personnel," pp. 167–71, lists the contents of sample kits of barefoot doctors. By the mid-1970s the training period for barefoot doctors had been extended from three or six months to a year. Marilynn M. Rosenthal and Jay R. Greiner, "The Barefoot Doctors of China: From Political Creation to Professionalization," *Human Organization* 41 (1982): 330–41, explore Mao's distrust of urban physicians and its role in the creation of the barefoot doctor program. Geoffrey Sek Yiu Lieu, "Barefoot Doctors in the People's Republic of China: A Study of the Medical Auxiliary's Role in Rural Health Care Delivery" (master's thesis, Washington University, St. Louis, 1974), explores the contents of manuals prepared to train barefoot doctors.

50. Peter Kong-ming New and Mary Louie New, "Health Care in the People's Republic of China: The Barefoot Doctor," *Inquiry* 12, no. 2, supplement (1975): 103–13; Victor W. Sidel, "The Barefoot Doctors of the People's Republic of China," *New England Journal of Medicine* 286 (1972): 1292–1300; and Sidel, "Medical Personnel," 153–72. On women barefoot doctors, see "Barefoot Doctors Active in Rural Child Health Care," *Chinese Medical Journal* 1 (1975): 95–98.

51. Chen Haifeng, "Pharmaceuticals and Medical Apparatus," in *Modern Chinese Medicine,* vol. 3, *Chinese Health Care,* ed. Chen Haifeng and Zhu Chao (Lancaster: MTP Press, 1984), 280, reports rapid progress in building the capacity to manufacture Western medicines, including antibiotics, between the 1950s and 1982, but does not discuss quantities, timing, or specific medications. These volumes provide the official image of medicine and health care.

52. This is the argument made by Ruth Sidel and Victor W. Sidel, *The Health of China* (Boston: Beacon Press, 1982), esp. pp. 27–34. On health programs in the 1960s, see esp. Banister, *China's Changing Population,* pp. 61–62 and 85–88; Chen, *Medicine in Rural China,* esp. p. 66; Jon E. Rohde, "Health for All in China: Principles and Relevance for Other Countries," in *Practising Health for All,* ed. David Morley, Jon E. Rohde, and Glen Williams (Oxford: Oxford University Press, 1983), pp. 5–16; and Victor W. Sidel and Ruth Sidel, *Serve the People: Observations on Medicine in the People's Republic of China* (New York: Josiah Macy Jr. Foundation, 1973), esp. pp. 78–88.

53. Zheng Liu, *Mortality and Health Issues: Mortality Patterns and Trends of Population in China* (Bangkok: Economic and Social Commission for Asia and the Pacific, 1986), pp. 27–32, supplies statistics.

54. Naisu Zhu et al., "Factors Associated with the Decline of the Cooperative Medical System and Barefoot Doctors in Rural China," *Bulletin of the World Health Organization* 67 (1989): 431–41.

55. Suzanne Pepper, "Education for the New Order," in *The Cambridge History of China,* vol. 14, *The People's Republic,* part I: *The Emergence of Revolutionary China 1949–1965,* ed. Roderick MacFarquhar and John K. Fairbank (Cambridge: Cambridge University Press, 1987), pp. 186 and 207–17; and K. E. Priestley, "Education in the People's Republic of China: Beginnings," in *Education and Communism in China: An Anthology of Commentary and Documents,* ed. Stewart E.

Fraser (London: Pall Mall Press, 1971), pp. 53–61. On the teacher shortage, see Leo A. Orleans, "Quality of Education," in *Education and Communism in China,* pp. 82–85; and on the period 1958–65, see Suzanne Pepper, "New Directions in Education," in *People's Republic,* pp. 398–431.

56. Vilma Seeberg, *Literacy in China: The Effect of the National Development Context and Policy on Literacy Levels, 1949–79* (Bochum, Germany: Brockmeyer, 1990), pp. 265–66 and 268.

57. World Bank, *World Development Indicators 2004 on CD-ROM* (Washington: World Bank, 2004).

58. Glen Peterson, *The Power of Words: Literacy and Revolution in South China, 1949–95* (Vancouver: University of British Columbia Press, 1997), pp. 3–6, summarizes scholarly judgments, proposes a favorable view of efforts to improve literacy in the Maoist era, and then does not express an opinion about the literacy level or trend in the period 1956–70. Peterson (pp. 6–16) also recognizes efforts to build population literacy in the decades preceding 1949. Peter J. Seybolt, *Revolutionary Education in China: Documents and Commentary* (White Plains, NY: International Arts and Sciences Press, 1973), discusses many things impeding gains in education and literacy in the later 1950s and 1960s, among them repeated but usually vague changes in policy direction from Beijing.

59. Gail Henderson and Myron S. Cohen, *The Chinese Hospital: A Socialist Work Unit* (New Haven: Yale University Press, 1984), describe the operation of the danwei to which they were attached in 1979–80, discuss the cost of medical care, and compare circumstances in peasant communes and other parts of the Chinese system. Victor N. Shaw, *Social Control in China: A Study of Chinese Work Units* (Westport, CT: Praeger, 1996), describes the system in the period 1979–94, but gives little information about health.

60. On mortality during the period of economic reforms, see Christopher Grigoriou, Patrick Guillaumont, and Wenyan Yang, "Child Mortality under Chinese Reforms," *China Economic Review* 16 (2005): 441–64.

61. World Bank, *China: Long-Term Issues and Options in the Health Transition* (Washington: World Bank, 1992), surveys the cause of death profile in 1986. The essays in Alan R. Hinman et al., eds., *Health Services in Shanghai County,* supplement to no. 9 of *American Journal of Public Health* 72 (1982), provide details about the system in one county in 1980 and on achievements in health since 1950. China Health Care Study Group, *Health Care in China: An Introduction* (Geneva: Christian Medical Commission, 1974), p. 54, reports massive and sudden declines in mortality from tuberculosis, smallpox, typhoid fever, dysentery, and cholera between 1950 and 1956.

62. David Blumenthal and William Hsiao, "Privatization and Its Discontents—The Evolving Chinese Health Care System," *New England Journal of Medicine* 353 (Sept. 15, 2005): 1165–70. On the decline of barefoot doctors, see Jeffrey P. Koplan et al., "The Barefoot Doctor: Shanghai County Revisited," *American Journal of Public Health* 75 (1985): 768–70; and Zhu et al., "Factors Associated with the Decline." Some provinces preserved the system into the 1990s, while others dismantled it in the 1980s. Sydney D. White, "Deciphering 'Integrated Chinese and

Western Medicine' in the Rural Lijiang Basin: State Policy and Local Practice(s) in Socialist China," *Social Science and Medicine* 49 (1999): 1333–47, reports that the village doctors, the former barefoot doctors, continued into the 1990s to rely on well-worn copies of *A Barefoot Doctor's Manual* and on its herbal remedies. On health services in 1990 see Willy De Geyndt, Xiyan Zhao, and Shunli Liu, *From Barefoot Doctor to Village Doctor in Rural China* (Washington: World Bank, 1992).

63. On urban-rural disparities in health care and infant mortality, and the deterioration of rural health, see Leiyu Shi, "Health Care in China: A Rural-Urban Comparison after the Socioeconomic Reforms," *Bulletin of the World Health Organization,* 71 (1993): 723–36.

64. Survival improved again in the 1990s. See Judith Banister and Xiaobo Zhang, "China, Economic Development and Mortality Decline," *World Development* 33 (2005): 21–41; and Ian G. Cook and Trevor J. B. Drummer, "Changing Health in China: Re-evaluating the Epidemiological Transition Model," *Health Policy* 67 (2004): 329–43.

8. Oil-Rich Lands

1. United Nations, Demographic Yearbook: Historical Supplement 1948–1997 CD-ROM (New York: Department of Economic and Social Affairs, Statistical Office, United Nations, n.d.); and World Bank, *World Development Indicators 2004 on CD-ROM* (Washington: World Bank, 2004).

2. Paul W. Harrison, *Doctor in Arabia* (New York: Day, 1940), esp. pp. 126–27, 133–34. Trachoma is an eye infection associated with poverty, poor hygiene, and deficient supplies of water. It can be treated with antibiotics, but without treatment, repeated cases may lead to blindness.

3. Raymond O'Shea, *The Sand Kings of Oman* (London: Metheun, 1947), pp. 14 and 17. To the same effect, see Wendell Phillips, *Unknown Oman* (New York: D. McKay Co., 1966), esp. pp. 62–66.

4. Harrison, *Doctor in Arabia,* esp. pp. 31, 37, 131, 134, 291–92, and 301; and Phillips, *Unknown Oman,* pp. 80–82.

5. Robert Geran Landen, *Oman since 1856: Disruptive Modernization in a Traditional Arab Society* (Princeton: Princeton University Press, 1967), pp. 388, 407–9, and 422–24.

6. A U.S. survey in the mid-1950s made a rough estimate of the crude death rate at 60 per 1,000. See United Nations, *National Experience in the Formulation and Implementation of Population Policy, 1960–1976: Oman* (New York: United Nations, 1978), p. 3.

7. United Nations Development Programme, *Human Development Report 1998* (New York: Oxford University Press, 1998), p. 149; and World Bank, *World Development Indicators 2001* (Washington: World Bank, 2001), CD-ROM.

8. Miriam Joyce, *The Sultanate of Oman: A Twentieth-Century History* (Westport, CT: Praeger, 1995), esp. 52–59, 95–99, and 103–12.

9. Calvin H. Allen, Jr. and W. Lynn Rigsbee II, *Oman under Qaboos: From Coup*

to Constitution 1970–1996 (London: Frank Cass, 2000), pp. 24–25. On social services for the pastoralists, who, in recent decades, comprised about 7 percent of the population, see Dawn Chatty, *Mobile Pastoralists: Development Planning and Social Change in Oman* (New York: Columbia University Press, 1996).

10. Ian Skeet, *Muscat and Oman: The End of an Era* (London: Faber and Faber, 1974), pp. 31, 56–58, and 177; quote from p. 183. Skeet qualifies this observation, limiting it to coastal Omanis.

11. Calvin H. Allen, *Oman: The Modernization of the Sultanate* (Boulder. CO: Westview Press, 1987), p. 102; Joyce, *Sultanate of Oman*, p. 111; and Oman, Ministry of Development, Information and Documentation Center, *Statistical Yearbook 1994* (Muscat: The Council, 1994), pp. 528 and 569.

12. UN estimates indicate that Kuwait added to survival at a pace of 1.5 years gain per year of calendar time in the late 1960s, the next fastest pace estimated for any country in any period.

13. Allan G. Hill and Lincoln C. Chen, *Oman's Leap to Good Health: A Summary of Rapid Health Transition in the Sultanate of Oman* (Muscat: n.p., 1996), p. 16. Allan Hill graciously provided me a copy of this book. World Bank, *World Development Indicators 2004*, first reports the level of health spending in Oman for 1997, when it was 229 current (1997) US dollars.

More detail on the development of health services may be found in A. G. Hill, A. Z. Muyeed, and J. A. al-Lawati, eds., *The Mortality and Health Transition in Oman: Patterns and Processes* (Muscat: n.p., 2000). Both Hill and Chen and Hill, Muyeed, and al-Lawati deal only with Omani citizens. The results of a UNICEF-sponsored study of health services and infant and child health may be found at www.unicef.org/evaldatabase/index_14179.html. However, when accessed October 22, 2004, that file was defective, excluding part of chapter 4 and all of chapter 5.

See also Nadeya Sayed Ali Mohammed, *Population and Development of the Arab Gulf States: The Case of Bahrain, Oman and Kuwait* (Aldershot, Hampshire: Ashgate, 2003), esp. 88–110; Richard Smith, "Oman: Leaping Across the Centuries," *British Medical Journal* 297 (1988): 540–44; and Onn Winckler, "Demographic Developments and Policies in the Arabian Gulf: The Case of Oman under Sultan Qabus," *Journal of South Asian and Middle Eastern Studies* 24 (2001): 34–60.

14. Murtadha J. Suleiman, Ahmed Al-Ghassany, and Samir Farid, *Oman Child Health Survey* (Muscat: Ministry of Health, 1992), as of 1988–89. Also Tom Gabriel, "Rural Change in the Sultanate of Oman: Social Organisation in the Wahiba Sands Region," *Asian Affairs* 19 (1988): 154–63, on rapid development in a rural area, including development of a cash economy.

15. Suleiman et al., *Oman Child Health Survey*, p. 43. J. S. Birks and C. A. Sinclair, "Successful Education and Human Resource Development—the Key to Sustained Economic Growth," in *Oman: Economic, Social and Strategic Developments*, ed. B. R. Pridham (London: Croom Helm, 1987), pp. 145–67, provides details about the education system in the 1970s and early 1980s.

16. Hill and Chen, *Oman's Leap*, p. 6.

17. Ibid., quote from p. 29.

18. There is also some conflict between descriptive accounts in the post-1970 period and claims of rapid and general improvement. See, for example, Fredrik Barth, *Sohar: Culture and Society in an Omani Town* (Baltimore: Johns Hopkins University Press, 1983), who in 1974–76 interviews and observations in the third largest city in Oman saw motor vehicles, generators, and pumps but no electricity, no piped water, and no arrangements for sewage disposal.

19. Hill et al., *Mortality and Health Transition in Oman,* pp. 3.1–3.37.

20. Jill Crystal, *Kuwait: The Transformation of an Oil State* (Boulder, CO: Westview Press., 1992), pp. 23–24 and 56–62; and Peter Mansfield, *Kuwait: Vanguard of the Gulf* (London: Hutchinson, 1990), pp. 91 and 94–100.

21. Allan G. Hill, "The Demography of the Kuwaiti Population of Kuwait," *Demography* 12 (1975): 537–48.

22. Note that a 1963 WHO report estimated life expectancy in Saudi Arabia at not greater than 30 years. See R. McGregor, "Saudi Arabia: Population and the Making of a Modern State," in *Populations of the Middle East and North Africa: A Geographical Approach,* ed. John Innes Clarke and W. B. Fisher (New York: Africana Pub. Corp., 1972), pp. 220–41.

23. On mortality in Iraq during the 1990s, see Mohamed M. Ali, John Blacker, and Gareth Jones, "Annual Mortality Rates and Excess Deaths of Children under Five in Iraq, 1991–98," *Population Studies* 57 (2003): 217–26.

24. Documentation on Iran, Iraq, Kuwait, and Saudi Arabia is thinner than on Oman. The information that follows has been drawn from the following sources. On Saudi Arabia: C. K. Chu, S. K. Djazar, and M. H. Adham, *Report on a Health Survey of Saudi Arabia* (Alexandria: n.p., 1963); Osman A. M. Nour et al., "Rapid Decline in Infant and Child Mortality," *Annals of Saudi Medicine* 12 (1992): 565–70; Zohair A. Sebai, *Health in Saudi Arabia,* 2 vols. (Riyad: Tihama Publications, 1985–87). On Kuwait: K. L. Kohli and Musa'ad H. Al-Omaim, "Patterns and Trends in Causes of Death in Kuwait: A Low Mortality Advanced Arab Country," *International Population Conference Florence 1985,* 4 vols. (Liège: International Union for the Scientific Study of Population, 1985), 2: 443–56; M. Sivamurthy, and Fawzi G. Torki, "Trends and Differentials in Mortality in Kuwait 1965–70," in Cairo Demographic Centre Research Monograph Series No. 8, *Mortality Trends and Differentials in Some African and Asian Countries* (Cairo: The Centre, 1982), pp. 353–401. On Iran: Amir Arsalan Afkhami, "Iran in the Age of Epidemics: Nationalism and the Struggle for Public Health, 1889–1926" (PhD diss., Yale University, 2003); Akbar Aghajanian, "Population Change in Iran 1966–86: A Stalled Demographic Transition?" *Population and Development Review* 17 (1991): 703–15; Djamchid Behnam and Mehdi Amani, *La population de l'Iran: Monographie* ([Paris]: CICRED, 1974); J. Bharier, "A Note on the Population of Iran 1900–1966," *Population Studies* 22 (1968): 273–79; Djamchid A. Momeni, "The Population of Iran: A Dynamic Analysis" (PhD diss., University of Texas, 1970). On Iraq: United States, Surgeon-General's Office, *Medical and Sanitary Survey on Iraq* (Washington: n.p., 1958).

25. A. M. Bahri et al., *La population de l'Algérie* (n.p.: CICRED, 1974); Dominique Tabutin, *Mortalité infantile et juvenile en Algérie* (Paris: n.p., 1976); and

K. C. Zachariah, M. Al-Molla, and A. Al-Ayat, "Basic Demographic Measures of Algeria," in Cairo Demographic Centre, *Demographic Measures and Population Growth in Arab Countries* (Cairo: n.p., 1970), pp. 1–25. G. Negadi, D. Tabutin, and J. Vallin, "Situation démographique en Algérie," in *La population de l'Algérie,* ed. Bahri et al., p. 20, suggest that mortality declined from 1916 to 1920, but I read their CDR estimates to show variation up to the 1930s, then decline. Jacques Vallin, "La mortalité en Algérie," *Population* 30 (1975): 1023–45, finds that mortality may have declined from the 1910s to the 1930s and then fluctuated. Official statistics exist for mortality from 1901, but deaths were underregistered.

26. Kamel Kateb, "L'expérance de vie à la naissance et la surmortalité féminine en Algérie en 1954," *Population* 53 (1998): 1209–26.

27. Yves Lacoste and André Prénant, "Quelques données du probleme algerien," *Pensée* 67 (1956): 15–42.

28. The term "explosion" comes from Fatima-Zohra Oufriha, *Système de santé et population en Algérie* ([Alger]: Editions Anep, 2002), p. 74; details on facilities and personnel, pp. 74–75.

29. K. E. Vaidyanathan and Hussein Al-Baradie, "Trends and Differentials of Mortality in Algeria," in *Mortality Trends and Differentials in Some African and Asian Countries,* pp. 77–123, report illiteracy in 1966. They estimate life expectancy in 1948 at 38.0 years for females and 37.6 for males. On the democratization of schools, see Kamel Kateb, "Démographie et démocratisation de l'école en Algérie (1962–2000)," *Maghreb-Machrek* nos. 171–72 (2001): 89–89.

30. Mahmoud S. Abdou Issa "Estimation of Mortality Level in Libya: 1972," in *Mortality Trends and Differentials in Some African and Asian Countries,* pp. 163–223; and R. G. Hartley, "Libya: Economic Development and Demographic Responses," in *Populations of the Middle East and North Africa: A Geographical Approach,* ed. John Innes Clarke and W. B. Fisher (New York: Africana Pub. Corp., 1972), pp. 315–47.

31. Hassan M. Ben-Taher, "The Planning and Design of Health Care Systems in Developing Countries: Case Study Libya" (master's thesis, University of Texas at Austin, 1980), reports statistics on health facilities and personnel from 1969 to 1977, and on school enrollments from 1958 to 1976.

32. See Abdel Momin Farag El-Fiki, "The Development of University Education in the Socialist People's Libyan Arab Jamahiriya: 1955 to 1980" (PhD diss., University of Oregon, 1982), pp. 108–36, on primary education in the period 1952–69.

33. Nigel Ash, *Libya: Education, Health and Housing* (London: Hakima PR, 1981), pp. 5, 8, 15, and 23–27.

34. Jorge Salazar-Carrillo and Bernadette West, *Oil and Development in Venezuela during the Twentieth Century* (Westport, CT: Praeger, 2004), p. 58, trace the early rise of oil revenues.

35. Ricardo Archila, *Historia de la sanidad en Venezuela,* 2 vols. (Caracas: Impr. Naciónal, 1956), 1: 188.

36. The sequence of legislation can be followed in Anibal R. Martinez, *Chronology of Venezuelan Oil* (London: Allen & Unwin, 1969).

37. Charles Rollins, "Raw Materials Development and Economic Growth: A Study of Bolivian and Venezuelan Experience" (PhD diss., Stanford University, 1956), esp. pp. 233, 350–59, investigated government spending from oil revenues across the period 1918 to 1954. Miriam Kornblith and Thais Maingón, *Estado y gasto público en Venezuela, 1936–1980* (Caracas: Universidad Central de Venezuela, 1985), pp. 58–60, continue the spending series from 1936–37 to 1980.

38. Terry Lynn Karl, *The Paradox of Plenty: Oil Booms and Petro-States* (Berkeley: University of California Press, 1997), deems Venezuela a petro-state, explores economic deterioration and political decay, and associates the country with other oil states held to have failed, including Algeria, Indonesia, Iran, and Nigeria. Her full list of petro-states appears on p. 17.

39. Ana Teresa Guitiérrez, "La búsqueda de una ilusión: La investigación sobre malaria en Venezuela," *Quipu* 8 (1991): 171–200.

40. Arturo Luis Bertí and José Antonio Jove, "Saneamiento en el medio rural," in *III Congreso medico social panamericano, Caracas, Marzo 1951* (Caracas: n.p., 1951), p. 209.

41. Archila, *Historia de la sanidad,* esp. 1: 181–84, 211, 217, and the discussion continues through volume 2; Bertí and Jove, "Saneamiento en el medio rural," 208–98, with photographs of equipment, construction, latrines, and other innovations; and R. B. Hill and E. I. Benarroch, *Anquilostomiasis y paludismo en Venezuela* (Caracas: Editorial Elite, 1940), which details the collection of information about hookworm and malaria, early efforts to combat those diseases, and the 1927 campaign in the Maracay region, also with photographs. See also José Gregorio Brito Campos, "Tratamientos antihelmínticos para el control de la anquilostomiasis en Venezuela (1927–1941)," in *Historia, salud y sociedad en Venezuela,* ed. Germán Yépez Colmenares (Caracas: Presidencia de la República: Fondo Naciónal de Ciencia, Tecnología e Innovación, Instituto de Estudios Hispanoamericanos, 2002), pp. 191–95; Rigel Ochoa Molina, "Las campaña proletrinas y su alcance sanitario durante la Venezuela gomecista," in *Historia, salud y sociedad,* pp. 123–41; and, on malaria, Omar Roa Véliz, "La comisíon Rockefeller y la malaria en Maracay entre 1927 y 1930," in *Historia, salud y sociedad,* pp. 197–213.

42. Manuel A. Donís Ríos, "Aproximación al estudio de la mortalidad infantil en Venezuela entre 1920 y 1935," *Boletin de la Academia Naciónal de la Historia* 71 (1988): 775–90. On earlier sanitary reforms in Caracas, especially from 1890 to 1910, see Arturo Almandoz, "The Shaping of Venezuelan Urbanism in the Hygiene Debate of Caracas, 1880–1910," *Urban Studies* 37 (2000): 2073–89.

43. Archila, *Historia de la sanidad,* 1: 265ff., 383–84, and 2: 33 and 289–90.

44. Aureo Yepéz Castillo, "La relación entre el crecimiento demográfico y la inscripción escolar en primaria en el periodo 1873–1950 en Venezuela," *Boletin de la Academia Naciónal de la Historia* 69 (1986): 443–59.

45. Pan American Health Organization, *Health Conditions in the Americas 1977–1980* (Washington: Pan American Health Organization, 1982), p. 161.

46. José Miguel Avilán Rovira et al., "Evolución de las condiciónes de salud (1936–1985): Indicadores de salud y bienestar," *VII Congreso Venezolano de salud*

pública, 7 vols. (Caracas: La Biblioteca, 1987), 1: 95–231, relying on diagnosed cases, which in 1940 comprised 59 percent of deaths. José Miguel Avilán Rovira, "Situación de salud en Venezuela según las estadísticas de mortalidad 1940–1995," *Gaceta médica de Caracas* 106 (1998): 169–96, updates coverage. See also Isabel Licha, "El impacto modernizador de la ingenieria sanitaria en Venezuela: El caso del INOS y de otras instituciónes sanitarias," *Quipu* 6 (1989): 217–36.

47. Peter Lindert, "The Rise of Social Spending, 1880–1930," *Explorations in Economic History* 31 (1994): 1–37; and Lindert, *Growing Public: Social Spending and Economic Growth since the Eighteenth Century,* 2 vols. (Cambridge: Cambridge University Press, 2004), esp. 1: 20–21, 171–90. Lindert draws evidence from several countries in western Europe plus Australia, Canada, Greece, Japan, New Zealand, and the United States. He defines social spending (1: 6) to include public spending on public health and education, but not specifically on health care, plus poor relief and family assistance, unemployment compensation, publicly funded pensions, and housing subsidies.

9. The Latin American Case: Mexico

1. G. B. Rodgers, "Income and Inequality as Determinants of Mortality: An International Cross-Section Analysis," *Population Studies* 33 (1979): 343–51.

2. For crude death rates in the late nineteenth century see Edmundo M. Narancio, Federico Capurro Calamet, and Agustin Ruano Fournier, *Historia y análisis estadístico de la población del Uruguay* (Montevideo: Peña & Co., 1939), p. 238; and Juan Rial Roade, *Población y desarrollo de un pequeño pais: Uruguay 1830–1930* (Montevideo: Centro de Informaciónes y Estudios del Uruguay, 1983), p. 122.

3. However, short-run variations in economic conditions in the period 1920–70 did show quite small effects on infant and non-infant mortality. See Alberto Palloni, Kenneth Hill, and Guido Pinto Aguirre, "Economic Swings and Demographic Changes in the History of Latin America," *Population Studies* 50 (1996): 105–32.

4. Samuel Morley, *The Income Distribution Problem in Latin America and the Caribbean* (Santiago: ECLAC, 2001), p. 10, from José Antonio Ocampo's introduction, and pp. 15–18.

5. Zadia M. Feliciano, "Mexico's Demographic Transformation: From 1900 to 1990," in *A Population History of North America,* ed. Michael R. Haines and Richard H. Steckel (Cambridge: Cambridge University Press, 2000), pp. 601–30, quote from p. 615. Mexico's gross domestic product rose rapidly from the early 1920s through the 1970s, excepting only the early 1930s; see Francisco Alba, *The Population of Mexico: Trends, Issues, and Policies* (New Brunswick, NJ: Transaction Books, 1982), pp. 93–95.

6. Miguel E. Bustamante, "La coordinación de los servicios sanitarios federales y locales como factor de progreso higiénico en México," in *La atención médica rural en México 1930–1980,* ed. Héctor Hernández Llamas (Mexico City: Instituto Mexicano del Seguro Social, 1984), pp. 35–90, esp. 43–49. Nathan L. Whetten,

"Salud y mortalidad en el México rural," in *La atención medica rural en México,* pp. 147–79, reports on causes of death in the period 1938–42. Official statistics understate mortality throughout 1922–60; see Eduardo Cordero, "La subestimación de la mortalidad infantil en México," *Demografía y economía,* 2 (1968): 44–62. The causes of death that Bustamente lists also dominated the profile of deaths in Mexico City in the period 1904–12 as reported in Alberto J. Pani, *Hygiene in Mexico: A Study of Sanitary and Educational Problems,* trans. Ernest L. de Gogorza (New York: G. P. Putnam's Sons, 1917), pp. 191–99.

7. James Angus McLeod, "Public Health, Social Assistance and the Consolidation of the Mexican State: 1888–1940" (PhD diss., Tulane University, 1990), pp. 115–16. That was also Pani's argument in *Hygiene in Mexico,* esp. p. 171.

8. Louise Schoenhals, "Mexico Experiments in Rural and Primary Education: 1921–1930," *Hispanic American Historical Review* 44 (1964): 22–43; see p. 34.

9. Anthony J. Mazzaferri, "Public Health and Social Revolution in Mexico: 1877–1930" (PhD diss., Kent State University, 1968), pp. 181–86; Ramón Eduardo Ruiz, *Mexico: The Challenge of Poverty and Illiteracy* (San Marino, CA: Huntington Library, 1963); Schoenhals, "Mexico Experiments in Rural and Primary Education," pp. 22–43; and Mary Kay Vaughan, *The State, Education, and Social Class in Mexico, 1880–1928* (DeKalb: Northern Illinois University Press, 1982), esp. pp. 127–64 and 185–85.

10. James Wallace Wilkie, *The Mexican Revolution: Federal Expenditure and Social Change since 1910,* 2nd ed., rev. (Berkeley: University of California Press, 1970), pp. 160–61.

11. Elaine Cantrell Lacy, "Literacy Policies and Programs in Mexico, 1920–1958" (Ph. D. diss., Arizona State University, 1991), pp. 88 and 100 n. 62.

12. Mary Kay Vaughan, *Cultural Politics in Revolution: Teachers, Peasants, and Schools in Mexico, 1930–1940* (Tucson: University of Arizona Press, 1997), pp. 32 and 59.

13. McLeod, "Public Health," p. 117. However, John Steinbeck, *The Forgotten Village* (New York: Viking Press, 1941), describes continuing reluctance to accept medical and public health innovations in a village meant to typify common experience.

14. Margaret E. Leahy, *Development Strategies and the Status of Women: A Comparative Study of the United States, Mexico, the Soviet Union, and Cuba* (Boulder, CO: L. Rienner Publishers, 1986), pp. 47–64, quote from p. 62.

15. Wilkie, *Mexican Revolution,* pp. 164–68.

16. Anne-Emanuelle Birn, "Local Health and Foreign Wealth: The Rockefeller Foundation's Public Health Programs in Mexico, 1924–1951" (PhD diss., Johns Hopkins University, 1993), p. 79 for quote, and esp. 77–95.

17. Alba, *Population of Mexico,* pp. 39–42.

18. Anna Maria Kapelusz-Poppi, "Physician Activists and the Development of Rural Health in Postrevolutionary Mexico," *Radical History Review* 80 (2001): 35–50, quote from p. 36.

19. Alba, *Population of Mexico,* pp. 97–99.

20. Claudia Agostoni, *Monuments of Progress: Modernization and Public Health*

in Mexico City, 1876–1910 (Calgary: University of Calgary Press, 2003), pp. 117–53; and Mazzaferri, "Public Health and Social Revolution in Mexico," pp. 289–92.

21. McLeod, "Public Health," pp. 189–90.

22. Alejandro Mina Valdés, "La medición indirecta de la mortalidad infantil y en los primeros años de vida en México," in *La mortalidad en México: Niveles, tendencies y determinantes,* ed. Mario Bronfman and José Gómez de Léon (Mexico City: El Colegio de México, Centro de Estudios Demográficos y de Desarrollo Urbano, 1988), pp. 273–306.

23. James J. Horn, "The Mexican Revolution and Health Care, or the Health of the Mexican Revolution," *Latin American Perspectives* 10 (1983): 24–39.

24. Rosario Cardenas and Patricia Fernández Ham, "Características de la mortalidad en México: Tendencias recientes y perspectivas," in *La población de México al final del siglo XX,* ed. Héctor Hiram Hernández Bringas and Catherine Menkes (Mexico City: Sociedad Mexicana de Demografía, 1998), pp. 45–66.

10. Fecal Disease, Malaria, and Tuberculosis

1. Richard G. Feachem et al., *Sanitation and Disease: Health Aspects of Excreta and Wastewater Management* (New York: Wiley, 1983), pp. 9–16 for a summary, and passim for detailed discussions of individual pathogens and diseases.

2. League of Nations, Health Organisation, *Report on an Investigation into the Sanitary Conditions in Persia undertaken on Behalf of the Health Committee of the League of Nations at the Request of the Persian Government* (Geneva: Imp. Atar, 1925), pp. 36–37, 43, 50, and 57; and Rosalie Slaughter Morton, *A Doctor's Holiday in Iran,* rev. ed. (New York: Funk & Wagnalls Co., 1940), esp. pp. 50, 52, 208. Both sources report that the Anglo-Iranian Oil Company first introduced sanitary improvements, such as the chlorination of water, in the province where it was operating.

3. B. E. Washburn, *The Health Game* (London: Churchill, 1930), pp. 12–13. Washburn reprinted material from *Jamaica Public Health* in this collection.

4. James C. Riley, *Poverty and Life Expectancy: The Jamaica Paradox* (Cambridge: Cambridge University Press, 2005), esp. pp. 82–91, provides extensive detail on the hookworm campaign and on declining mortality from fecal disease.

5. Rockefeller Archive Center, Record Group 2, 462, box 10, folder 85, Jacocks to Victor G. Heiser, June 6, 1928.

6. Rockefeller Archive Center, Record Group 12.1, Victor G. Heiser diaries, IV, 179.

7. See W. W. Cort et al., *Studies on Hookworm, Ascaris and Trichuris in Panama* (Baltimore: Johns Hopkins University, School of Hygiene and Public Health, 1929), pp. 88–89, for a description of fecal pollution before the U.S. campaign began.

8. Brent H. Hoff, *Mapping Epidemics: A Historical Atlas of Disease* (New York: Franklin Watts, [2000]), p. 57, gives a map showing the global distribution of malaria around 1850.

9. Leonard Jan Bruce-Chwatt and Julian de Zulueta, *The Rise and Fall of Malaria in Europe: A Historico-Epidemiological Study* (Oxford: Oxford University Press, 1980), esp. pp. 6–7; and Erwin H. Ackerknecht, *Malaria in the Upper Mississippi Valley, 1760–1900* (Baltimore: Johns Hopkins Press, 1945), pp. 62–101.

10. Margaret Humphreys, *Malaria: Poverty, Race, and Public Health in the United States* (Baltimore: Johns Hopkins University Press, 2001), pp. 39–40, regarding the Upper Mississippi Valley. Humphreys (pp. 110–12) provides evidence of migration out of malarial areas in the American South in the late 1930s and suggests that earlier migrations may help explain the nineteenth-century retreat of malaria in the American Midwest.

11. Gordon Harrison, *Mosquitoes, Malaria and Man: A History of the Hostilities since 1880* (New York: Dutton, 1978), pp. 125–40 and 169–70.

12. Richard Johnson, "Malaria and Malaria Control in the USSR, 1917–1941" (PhD diss., Georgetown University, 1988), p. 215. Mary Schaeffer Conroy, "Malaria in Late Tsarist Russia," *Bulletin of the History of Medicine* 56 (1982): 41–55, also discusses malaria incidence.

13. Edwin R. Nye and Mary E. Gibson, *Ronald Ross, Malariologist and Polymath: A Biography* (New York: St. Martin's Press, 1997), pp. 238, 241, and 248. Contrast this with practice in the Soviet Union, described by Johnson, "Malaria and Malaria Control in the USSR," pp. 196 and 201.

14. A. A. Sandosham, *Malariology, with Special Reference to Malaya* (Singapore: University of Malaya Press, 1959), esp. pp. 18, 25, 249, provides valuable information about control techniques. Malcolm Watson, "Some Pages from the History of the Prevention of Malaria [part 2]," *Glasgow Medical Journal* 123 (1935): 130–53, reports his discovery that frequent application of a mixture of mineral oils would control mosquitoes even in fast-moving streams.

15. Bruce-Chwatt and Zulueta, *Rise and Fall of Malaria,* p. 154; and Johnson, "Malaria and Malaria Control in the USSR," p. 222. That trend was reversed during World War II, but resumed after the war with DDT use.

16. Malcolm Watson, *The Prevention of Malaria in the Federated Malay States: A Record of Twenty Years' Progress,* 2nd ed. (London: J. Murray, 1921); see, e.g., pp. 9–20 on the town of Klang. Also Ronald Ross, *Report on the Prevention of Malaria in Mauritius* (London: n.p., 1908), which reveals Ross's plan for prevention; and Leonard J. Bruce-Chwatt and Joan M. Bruce-Chwatt, "Malaria in Mauritius: As Dead as the Dodo," *Bulletin of the New York Academy of Medicine,* 2nd Series, 50 (1974): 1069–80, on the success of the Ross program at reducing malaria incidence.

17. Paris green had been used in the 1880s and 1890s as an insecticide to protect crops from beetles, so it was not a new compound. James C. Whorton, "Insecticide Spray Residues and Public Health: 1865–1938," *Bulletin of the History of Medicine* 45 (1971): 219–41.

18. Vartan M. Amadouny, "The Campaign against Malaria in Transjordan, 1926–1946: Epidemiology, Geography, and Politics," *Journal of the History of Medicine and Allied Sciences* 52 (1997): 453–84; Nancy Elizabeth Gallagher, *Egypt's Other Wars: Epidemics and the Politics of Public Health* (Syracuse, NY: Syracuse University Press, 1990), p. 93; and Harrison, *Mosquitoes, Malaria and Man,* p. 187. Also

Hughes Evans, "European Malaria Policy in the 1920s and 1930s: The Epidemiology of Minutiae," *Isis* 80 (1989): 40–59.

19. Johnson, "Malaria and Malaria Control in the USSR," pp. 215–17.

20. Bruce-Chwatt and de Zulueta, *Rise and Fall of Malaria in Europe,* pp. 87 and 112; and Harrison, *Mosquitoes, Malaria and Man,* pp. 210–11.

21. Humphreys, *Malaria: Poverty, Race, and Public Health,* pp. 56–57.

22. Aviva Chomsky, *West Indian Workers and the United Fruit Company in Costa Rica, 1870–1940* (Baton Rouge: Louisiana State University Press, 1996), pp. 101–2, describes a cost-saving approach taken by the United Fruit Company, which eschewed both the use of quinine as a prophylactic and mosquito control at breeding sites in favor attacking mosquitoes in the living quarters of its workers and treating the sick. Malaria mortality nevertheless declined.

23. The problems of mosquito control differed appreciably from country to country, which is illustrated by V. R. Muraleeldharan and D. Veeraraghavan, "Anti-Malarial Policy in the Madras Presidency: An Overview of the Early Decades of the Twentieth Century," *Medical History* 36 (1992): 290–305; and Nancy Leys Stepan, "'The Only Serious Terror in These Regions': Malaria Control in the Brazilian Amazon," in *Disease in the History of Modern Latin America: From Malaria to AIDS,* ed. Diego Armus (Durham, NC: Duke University Press, 2003), pp. 25–50.

24. The first synthetic quinine was introduced in 1891, but it was 1934 before a synthetic superior to natural quinine was found. Mark Honigsbaum, *The Fever Trail: In Search of the Cure for Malaria* (New York: Farrar, Straus & Giroux, 2002), pp. 217–18.

25. Joel G. Breman, Martin S. Alilio, and Anne Mills, "Conquering the Intolerable Burden of Malaria: What's New, What's Needed, A Summary," *American Journal of Tropical Medicine and Hygiene* 71, supplement 2 (2004): 1–15; and L. Riopel, "Analysis of Pharmaceutical Development Issues for Malaria as Basis for Priority Setting," background paper, Oct. 18, 2004, Medicines for Malaria Venture, at mednet3.who.int/prioritymeds/report/background/malaria.doc, accessed May 30, 2006.

26. Amy L. Fairchild and Gerald M. Oppenheimer, "Public Health Nihilism vs. Pragmatism: History, Politics, and the Control of Tuberculosis," *American Journal of Public Health* 88 (1998): 1105–17; and Leonard G. Wilson, "The Historical Decline of Tuberculosis in Europe and America: Its Causes and Significance," *Journal of the History of Medicine and Allied Sciences* 45 (1990): 366–96. See also the exchange between Linda Bryder and Wilson in *Journal of the History of Medicine and Allied Sciences* 46 (1991): 358–68. On the role of protein in resistance to tuberculosis, see William D. Johnston, "Tuberculosis," in *The Cambridge World History of Human Disease,* ed. Kenneth F. Kiple (Cambridge: Cambridge University Press, 1993), p. 1061.

27. By 1906 Koch was promoting isolation as the best technique for tuberculosis control. See Linda Bryder, *Below the Magic Mountain: A Social History of Tuberculosis in Twentieth-Century Britain* (Oxford: Clarendon Press, 1988), p. 30.

28. The following studies have been useful for this summary of experience with tuberculosis in the West: Barbara Bates, *Bargaining for Life: A Social History of*

Tuberculosis, 1876–1938 (Philadelphia: University of Pennsylvania Press, 1992), who deals mostly with Pennsylvania; Bryder, *Below the Magic Mountain;* Georgina D. Feldberg, *Disease and Class: Tuberculosis and the Shaping of Modern North American Society* (New Brunswick, NJ: Rutgers University Press, 1995); Isabelle Grellet and Caroline Kruse, *Histoires de la tuberculose: Les fièvres de l'âme 1800–1940* (Paris: Editions Ramsay, 1983); and F. B. Smith, *The Retreat of Tuberculosis 1850–1950* (London: Croom Helm, 1988).

29. George Borodin, *Red Surgeon* (London: Museum Press, 1944), p. 40; and Edward Podolsky, *Red Miracle: The Story of Soviet Medicine* (New York: Beechhurst, 1947), pp. 85–88.

30. Sherwood Hall, *With Stethoscope in Asia* (McLean, VA: MCL Associates, 1978), p. 436, reports the introduction of Christmas seals in Korea in 1932, taken from the U.S. model.

31. William Johnston, *The Modern Epidemic: A History of Tuberculosis in Japan* (Cambridge, MA: Council on East Asian Studies, Harvard University, 1995), p. 91, reports that mortality from tuberculosis declined during 1919–33 but rose from 1933 until after World War II. Johnston (p. 103) suggests that sanatoria and attempts to educate the populace about this disease were not enough to diminish mortality.

32. Michael Zdenek David, "The White Plague in the Red Capital: The Control of Tuberculosis in Moscow, 1900–1940" (MD thesis, Yale University, 2001), esp. pp. 339–403 and figure 5.1.

33. Diego Armus, "Tango, Gender, and Tuberculosis in Buenos Aires, 1900–1940," in *Disease in the History of Modern Latin America: From Malaria to AIDS,* ed. Diego Armus (Durham, NC: Duke University Press, 2003), p. 123; and Ruben Gorlero Bacigalupi, *Historia de la lucha antituberculosa en el Uruguay* (n.p.: n.p., 1964), pp. 172–73.

34. Riley, *Poverty and Life Expectancy,* esp. pp. 39–46, 97–101.

35. H. Hyslop Thomson, *Consumption: Its Prevention and Home Treatment: A Guide for the Use of Patients* (London: H. Frowde, 1910), quotes from p. 11.

36. Thomas Dormandy, *The White Death: A History of Tuberculosis* (New York: New York University Press, 2000), p. 174.

37. S. Adolphus Knopf, *Tuberculosis: A Preventable and Curable Disease: Modern Methods for the Solution of the Tuberculosis Problem* (New York: Moffat, Yard, 1909), pp. ix–x and 3–28 in particular. Information about later editions of this and the 1901 *Tuberculosis as a Disease of the Masses* has been obtained from a WorldCat search.

38. However, René J. Dubos and Jean Dubos, *The White Plague: Tuberculosis, Man and Society* (Boston: Little, Brown, 1952), pp. 211–15, review contributions to home treatment, beginning with an 1889 leaflet by Hermann Biggs with the title *Rules to Be Observed for the Prevention of the Spread of Consumption.* (This leaflet is reproduced in Thomas M. Daniel, *Captain of Death: The Story of Tuberculosis* [Rochester, NY: University of Rochester Press, 1997], p. 89.) Dormandy, *The White Death,* p. 297, dismisses any benefits from learning how to detect tuberculosis in others.

39. In Korea Sherwood Hall, a U.S.-educated physician serving as a medical missionary, opened a sanatorium in 1928 and made home treatment advice part of the regimen. Hall, *With Stethoscope in Asia,* esp. pp. 387, 421.

40. See the set of four pamphlets written by Dorothy Deming and distributed by the National Tuberculosis Association under the general title *Home Care of Tuberculosis: The Family Physician in Charge; A Guide for the Family; Hints for the Patient;* and *Pointers for Nurses.* All four were published in New York in 1943 by the National Tuberculosis Association.

41. I. Lazarevich, *La médecine en U.R.S.S.* (Paris: Les Iles d'or, 1953), pp. 61–62.

42. The quote is from Borodin, *Red Surgeon,* p. 38, citing a slogan used in the Soviet Union around 1939.

Conclusion

1. See e.g., United Nations, *Report on International Definition and Measurement of Standards and Levels of Living* (New York: United Nations, 1954).

2. See the UN publications *Declaration on Social Progress and Development* (New York: United Nations Office of Public Information, 1970); *Overcoming Obstacles to Institutional Development in the Least Developed Countries* (New York: United Nations, Department of International Economic and Social Affairs, 1991); and *Social Development: Advancing Social Development in a Globalizing World* (New York: United Nations, Department of Public Information, 2000).

3. Jennifer Prah Ruger, "The Changing Role of the World Bank in Global Health," *American Journal of Public Health* 95 (2005): 60–70.

4. Anne-Emanuelle Birn, "Gates's Grandest Challenge: Transcending Technology as Public Health Ideology," published online March 11, 2005 and available at image.thelancet.com/extras/04art6429web.pdf; and the Global Fund's *2004 Annual Report* at www.theglobalfund.org/en/files/Annual_Report_2004.pdf.

Index

Ackerknecht, Erwin H., 149

Africa, 15, 50; antibiotics and vaccines in, 46–48, 170; association of income and life expectancy in, 33; GDPpc in, 26; informal economy in, 25. *See also* North Africa; *specific countries*

Albania, 49, 100–102, 104, 108, 115, 152, 162, 166, 202n8; Soviet model in, 109

Al-Baradie, Hussein, 211n29

Algeria, 7, 15, 116, 119, 125–27, 131, 163, 212n38; development of oil reserves in, 117

Anglo-Iran Oil Company, 215n2

antibiotics, 4, 11, 46–48, 142, 143, 159, 170; in China, 111, 206n51; in Costa Rica, 84, 87; in Cuba, 93; in Jamaica, 95, 96; in Japan, 58; in Korea, 62

Arab nationalism, 119

Argentina, 5, 29, 133–36

Asia, 15, 50, 163, 169; antibiotics and vaccines in, 46–48, 170; sanitary improvements in, 144, 145. *See also specific countries*

Atkinson, Anthony, 60

Australia, 8, 9, 26, 185n2, 213n47

Avilán, José, 130

bacille Calmette-Guérin (BCG) vaccine, 58, 111, 129

Bahrain, 49

Banister, Judith, 110, 204n38

Barbados, 6, 50, 77

barefoot doctors, 5, 111, 112, 114

Barth, Fredrik, 210n18

Batista, Fulgencio, 88

Battista Grassi, Giovanni, 149

Belgium, 1, 7

Ben-Taher, Hassan M., 211n31

beriberi, 55

Bertí, Arturo Luis, 129

Betancourt, José F., 199n20

Biesanz, John, 76, 196n6

Biesanz, Mavis, 76, 196n6

Biggs, Hermann, 218n38

Bilharzia. *See* schistosomiasis

Bixby, Luis Rosero, 79

blacks, 186n6; Cuban, 92, 93, 98; Jamaican, 89, 95, 157

Bolsheviks, 106

Botswana, 6, 276

Britain, 38, 65, 69, 81; economic growth in, 1, 2, 7, 8; Jamaica and, 88–89, 95, 97, 98, 145, 156, 164; Kuwait and, 123; Libya and, 128; Malaya and, 152; Oman and, 118, 119, 121; Sri Lanka and, 164; tuberculosis in, 154, 157–59

British Caribbean, 15, 20, 186n6, 199n1. *See also* Jamaica

Bruce-Chwatt, Leonard Jan, 149, 201n7

bubonic plague, 118, 124; vaccine against, 48

Buddhist Reform Movement, 69

Bulgaria, 29, 104

Burma, 66

Text and Display: Galliard
Compositor: Integrated Composition Systems
Indexer: Ruth Elwell
Printer and binder: Sheridan Books, Inc.